Advance praise for *Be Your Own Herbalist*

"*Be Your Own Herbalist* takes us through the history and folklore of the magnificent world of herbal medicine and all it has to offer. Dr. Michelle Schoffro Cook provides practical and valuable information on how to easily incorporate herbal medicine into your everyday life. Whether you are searching for home remedies for common ailments or are an herbal practitioner, this book will certainly be useful."

— Dr. Cobi Slater, PhD, DNM, RHT, RNCP, NNCP,
author of *The Ultimate Metabolic Plan* and
The Ultimate Hormone Balancing Guidebook

"*Be Your Own Herbalist* highlights common yet extraordinary healing plants that grow wild or that can be planted in your garden or found at your local farmers' market or grocery store. Michelle Schoffro Cook shares many wonderful recipes for nutritious, healthful foods and offers an essential guide for anyone who wants to bring the power of herbs into their life!"

— Beverley Gray, herbalist, natural health practitioner, and author of
The Boreal Herbal: Wild Food and Medicine Plants of the North

T0126081

BE YOUR OWN HERBALIST

Also by Michelle Schoffro Cook, PhD, DNM

PRINT BOOKS

Boost Your Brain Power in 60 Seconds: The 4-Week Plan
for a Sharper Mind, Better Memory, and Healthier Brain (Rodale)

The 4-Week Ultimate Body Detox Plan:
A Program for Greater Energy, Health, and Vitality (Wiley)

The Probiotic Promise:
Simple Steps to Heal Your Body from the Inside Out (Da Capo)

60 Seconds to Slim: Balance Your Body Chemistry to Burn Fat Fast (Rodale)

The Ultimate pH Solution: Balance Your Body Chemistry
to Prevent Disease and Lose Weight (HarperCollins)

Weekend Wonder Detox:
Quick Cleanses to Strengthen Your Body and Enhance Your Beauty (Da Capo)

E-BOOKS

Acid-Alkaline Food Chart

Cancer-Proof: All-Natural Solutions for Cancer Prevention and Healing

Everything You Need to Know about Healthy Eating

Healing Recipes

The Vitality Diet: 21 Days to a Leaner, Healthier,
Happier, More Energetic You

BE YOUR OWN HERBALIST

Essential Herbs for Health, Beauty, and Cooking

Michelle Schoffro Cook, PhD, DNM

Illustrations by Peggy Duke

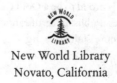

New World Library
Novato, California

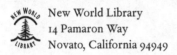

New World Library
14 Pamaron Way
Novato, California 94949

Illustrations by Peggy Duke (except p. 127)
Text design by Tona Pearce Myers

Library of Congress Cataloging-in-Publication Data
Names: Cook, Michelle Schoffro, author.
Title: Be your own herbalist : essential herbs for health, beauty, and cooking /
  Michelle Schoffro Cook, PhD, DNM.
Description: Novato, California : New World Library, [2016]
Identifiers: LCCN 2016003505 | ISBN 9781608684243 (paperback)
Subjects: LCSH: Herbs—Therapeutic use. | Cooking (Herbs) | Self-care,
  Health. | BISAC: HEALTH & FITNESS / Herbal Medications. | COOKING /
  Specific Ingredients / Herbs, Spices, Condiments. | GARDENING / Herbs. |
  COOKING / Health & Healing / General.
Classification: LCC RM666.H33 C685 2016 | DDC 615.3/21—dc23
LC record available at http://lccn.loc.gov/2016003505

First printing, April 2016
ISBN 978-1-60868-424-3
EISBN 978-1-60868-425-0
Printed in Canada on 100% postconsumer-waste recycled paper

New World Library is proud to be a Gold Certified Environmentally
Responsible Publisher. Publisher certification awarded by Green Press
Initiative. www.greenpressinitiative.org

10   9   8   7   6   5   4   3

I dedicate this book to the love of my life,
my husband, Curtis.
You are my inspiration in all that I do.
I am eternally grateful to share life with you, my soulmate.

Contents

Foreword

As clinical herbalists and founders of the Harmonic Arts Botanical Dispensary, we find Michelle Schoffro Cook's book to be in alignment with what we are facilitating in our company and practice: teaching people to be their own herbalists. This concept appeals to us in many ways: It takes the power of healing away from external entities and puts it back into the hands of each unique being to create their own story of health. It fosters the confidence to trust the body's innate wisdom in working with the therapeutic properties that plants have to offer. Most important, it allows the body to work within the natural scope of what Mother Nature intended, thus limiting the need for man-made, isolated chemical compounds in the form of pharmaceuticals and highly concentrated extracts. Foreign to the body's natural systems, these can create harmful side effects and addictive patterns.

We view the path of wellness as a way for each person to create their own adventure and design their unique lifestyle. Once a person is empowered with natural health knowledge and information, they can decipher what the best possible health choice is in any given moment. In a world full of health trends, it can be difficult to sort out what is what. Going back to basics and looking at what has healed people time and again throughout history and across a multitude of indigenous cultures brings tried-and-tested validity. By comparison, our modern allopathic medicine system is very young and limited in scope.

There is an important place for both herbal and modern medicine in the world. In this book, Dr. Cook clearly demonstrates the complementary nature of plants as health allies. Through our lifelong journeys of understanding health and wellness, we have come to recognize that what comes from the earth harmoniously aligns with our bodies, also of the earth.

In *Be Your Own Herbalist*, Dr. Cook not only explores traditional uses of herbs but also gives credence to current applications, skillfully weaving traditional herbalism with proven modern scientific methods. She offers up-to-date, scientifically validated findings of successful uses of plant medicine.

This book focuses on thirty-one medicinal plants that can be found across multiple bioregions and are readily available fresh or dried in health-food stores and other markets. Knowing these plants intimately is more useful than being superficially acquainted with the larger spectrum of plant medicine. This book guides you in exploring these thirty-one great plants in a multifaceted way, giving you the opportunity to build with each one the kind of relationship you'd have with a dear friend. It also allows you to work with the plants from the outside in, preparing the herbs in a myriad of ways, from creating body-care products that introduce the plant's properties to the frontlines of your system to cooking them and letting food be your medicine. Fun and varied herbal concoctions let you play in the kitchen and discover your favorite ways of creating wellness for yourself and loved ones.

The clear, simple, and direct communication style in which this book is written allows for a gentle, welcoming entry point into the realm of herbalism. It confers the sense that a nurturing, supportive figure is holding your hand as you learn to work with herbs. Dr. Cook does a great job of breaking herbalism down into tangible steps that allow you to start playing with plants confidently, right away. You don't have to be an expert to be an at-home, practical herbalist, and this book will show you how. We are delighted to introduce such a fine work that puts the power back into the people's hands, allowing them to maintain good health and vitality and cultivate longevity. We welcome you through the doors of herbalism, as you embark on an exciting, purposeful journey into the world of plant medicine. As Dr. Cook inspires you to live a healthy, balanced, whole life, may you also do the same for those in your life. Viva the herbal revolution!

— Angela and Yarrow Willard,
clinical herbalists and cofounders of the Harmonic Arts Botanical
Dispensary, Vancouver Island, British Columbia, Canada

PART 1

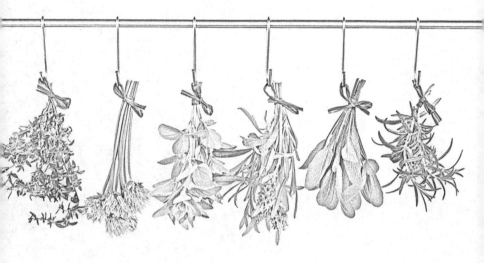

Everything You Need
to Get Started

1. Your Guide to Being Your Own Herbalist

I did not know that an uneventful spring day almost twenty-five years ago would become one of such significance in my life. I was nineteen and had just withdrawn from a university degree program in journalism because of severe illness. A few years earlier, my doctors had diagnosed a rare genetic disease. They proceeded to subject my body to harsh treatment that did nothing to alleviate the original symptoms but instead left me fragile, exhausted, and devastated as I watched my dreams and life fall apart. By the time I was nineteen, my life was not going as planned, but I had made peace with it.

On this particular spring day, I managed to get myself out of bed, washed, clothed, and onto the elevator, and even to take the fifty or so steps to sit on a park bench beside a nearby canal. Proud and exhausted from this unusual experience of getting myself outdoors, I was happy to sit in the sunlight and regain my breath. I was accustomed to spending the days alone in silence and contemplation: thinking and getting in touch with my feelings had replaced the physical activities that had once occupied my days.

I looked around and noticed that dotting the grass were clover leaves and their purple flowers, oddly shaped leaves that I later learned were lamb's quarters, and brilliant yellow dandelion heads. I wondered about the purpose of these plants, which gardeners seemed to hate so much. Only days earlier my doctor, who practiced hundreds of miles away, had told me over the phone that there really wasn't anything he could do to help me. He apologized with a sadness that seemed sincere and explained that the research on such a rare disease was antiquated at best. I had been hoping he would allay my fears and concerns about my health and a treatment that had produced side effects worse than the condition it was meant to treat. Instead, his words filled me with an overwhelming grief for the life I had once had and a hopelessness I never imagined possible.

Yet this particular combination of grief and hopelessness, experienced on this park bench on this particular day, would change my life. While contemplating the purpose of these odd herbal misfits in the monoculture we know as grass and at the same time knowing that the most caring physician of the dozens who treated me had given up any hope of improvement in my condition, I asked myself, "What if Mother Nature provided the cure for every disease imaginable? What if these plants that gardeners dismiss as weeds could heal a person's ills?" I felt the sunlight on my face and warming my body, and at that moment I knew that I needed to study herbs. I signed up for the only course I could find, a distance-learning course, in hopes that in the limited periods of lucidity I had each day, I could learn about herbal medicine.

That day marked the first step on a powerful and amazing journey that has lasted nearly twenty-five years. I hope that reading this book will help you take an important step on your own journey.

My study of Mother Nature's medicine, as I call it, has taken many forms. That first distance-education herbal course fueled a passion for herbs that led me to read endlessly and take additional courses. As my health improved, I was able to venture on guided herb walks and voraciously research the latest studies in herbal medicine.

I learned about plants that healed all sorts of diseases. "How could I not have been taught this before?" I thought, angry and hopeful both at once. I learned about plants that eliminated arthritis, those that reversed diabetes, and even plants that healed cancer. It seemed that for every illness, Mother Nature had a cure that outranked our best pharmaceutical medicine. Shockingly, many of these medicines go ignored, even though they lie right at our feet.

As I grew stronger, I began to drive out to the forest near my home, carrying the manual from my first herbal course along with a bag and scissors to collect these wild medicines. It was as though a magical kingdom had appeared before me. Every time I spotted a new flower or plant, I flipped through the pages of my well-worn textbook to find out what this overlooked plant could heal.

I discovered that the much-hated dandelion purifies the blood and kidneys and may even be a cancer cure. I found that calendula heals skin conditions, echinacea restores the immune system, feverfew banishes migraines, juniper heals the kidneys, milk thistle protects the liver, clover balances hormones, and St. John's wort lifts the spirits. The list went on. How could I have seen these plants on lawns, in forests, and along riverbeds as a child, yet never have learned of their amazing healing abilities? Spurred by my newfound knowledge and greatly improved health, I continued my studies to become a board-certified doctor of natural medicine, registered nutritional consulting practitioner, certified herbal medicine practitioner, and registered orthomolecular health specialist. As my health improved, my passion for and belief in the healing abilities of herbs grew stronger.

At the same time, I learned that billion-dollar pharmaceutical companies were getting rich scouring the earth for new plant compounds they could extract, synthesize, patent, and then manufacture into so-called wonder drugs that promise to reverse and even cure our worst ailments and diseases. But in separating these plant compounds from the essential nutrients and other beneficial substances found naturally alongside the original compound, and then attempting to re-create these naturally occurring compounds in the laboratory, they were actually reducing the effectiveness of the plant medicine and creating drugs that carried long lists of side effects and frequently a steep price tag. I learned that the third leading cause of death is the *correct* use of these drugs and that they kill hundreds of thousands of people every year.

I learned that pharmaceutical companies held patents on many once-natural but now synthetically derived drugs that frequently allowed them to charge sick people hundreds or even thousands of dollars each month. I realized that many of these people were losing their pensions, their hard-earned cash, and even their homes in a desperate attempt to recover some semblance of a normal life. Millions of people couldn't afford the drugs that they believed could restore their quality of life.

I knew that the medication I had been prescribed was killing me. I had all of the "common," "less common," and "rare" side effects and all but three of the "extremely rare" side effects listed in the pharmaceutical books for the drug I had been told my life depended on. The only three I hadn't experienced were blindness, coma, and death. More than a dozen specialists had told me I would surely die if I discontinued taking the medication. I decided that since they had been wrong about there being no hope for me, they were also wrong about the medication.

While my decision to discontinue the medication took only a second to make, it took me nearly two years to implement. Slowly and gradually I reduced my dose until, with bated breath, I took the last pill ...and waited...and waited...and waited. Finally, I had the evidence I needed to prove that my doctors, while well trained and mostly well intentioned, were wrong. Not only was I alive, but I felt hopeful again.

I'm not suggesting that there is no place for pharmaceutical drugs and so-called modern medicine in our society, but total reliance on this system is failing to help many people and actively ruining the lives of many others. It certainly has its strengths in emergency medicine, but at its core it has become a system that values profit over people, and that is something I cannot accept.

Conversely, Mother Nature's medicine, along with some expert guidance, can empower people, restore hope, and bring communities — poor or rich — together. Pharmaceutical-based medicine, due to its often-high cost, has frequently only been available to the rich, while natural medicine is available to rich and poor alike. Additionally, natural medicine is a local option that is readily available to people around the world, no matter how remote their communities may be. Pharmaceutical giants have largely played God by determining which diseases are worthy of their attention and research, decisions that are driven largely by profit. Conversely, there is no inherent bias in natural medicine. There are natural medicines for just about every condition that exists, and more applications are being discovered almost daily. Unlike many pharmaceutical drugs that kill or cause serious side effects even when they are correctly used, most natural medicines are safe when used correctly. Natural medicines are available to the suffering people who need them, regardless of their financial resources, their location in the world, or the type of disease from which they are suffering.

Every human being on the planet has a right to health. Herbs can offer the solution. They also offer the hope of relief from the widespread misery caused by unprecedented rates of serious and disabling diseases, from heart disease to diabetes, cancer, and HIV. Even when complete cures may not be possible, herbs can immensely improve a person's quality of life, as I know from experience. In the years since that spring day that changed my life, I have witnessed many people with debilitating and life-threatening illnesses restored to health, thanks to herbs and natural foods.

Herbs helped me rebuild my body, and while they have not undone all the damage caused by the injury I sustained from pharmaceutical-based medicine, I have lived more than two decades longer than many doctors predicted. I have also enjoyed a much better quality of life than I imagined possible that day on the park bench. Today I live with my husband on our property in the middle of the Coast Mountains in British Columbia, Canada. We grow a significant amount of our own food and herbs and live an increasingly self-sufficient life, independent of many of the corporations that now control the global food supply. We also strive to grow and make the natural medicines we need and use, independent of major drug companies.

I share this story with you not to discourage you from continuing any medical treatment you may be undergoing but to reinforce the healing power of herbal medicine. The choice I made was a personal one that was right for me; only you can decide whether the same choice is right for you.

In this book I want to share with you the exciting and empowering research on thirty-one common and accessible herbs, all of which are easy to grow and use daily as food and medicine. These herbs are among my favorites because they are indigenous to many places, readily available, easy to incorporate into food and body-care products, and powerfully therapeutic.

I am thrilled to share with you *Be Your Own Herbalist*, which instructs you on cultivating and using the world's oldest and most effective natural medicines. Throughout human history, we have relied on herbs in medicine. Only recently have we lost touch with these ancient healing agents in favor of drugs. Even though most of these compounds were originally derived from herbs, the process of isolating single compounds and synthesizing them in a laboratory results in harmful and sometimes life-threatening side effects. Most herbs contain dozens and sometimes even hundreds of healing compounds that work best (and cause the fewest side effects) in synergy. In many cases, the herbs are actually more effective than our best drug medicines. Of course, herbs are still medicine: we need to treat them with respect and recognize their potency. This also means learning how drug medicines might interact with herbal medicines and which herbs may not be right for everyone.

I understand from experience that exploring the realms of herbal medicine can be intimidating. After all, we've been taught that herbs are dangerous or inferior to pharmaceutical drugs. And that is one of the reasons I created this book: not only to impart the knowledge I have gained over the years but also to help you feel confident in using it to improve your health.

Additionally, over the years I could not find a single book that explained how to grow, cook with, and use herbs as food and medicine at home. Some books explain how to use herbs, others share information on how to grow them, and still others share the exciting research that proves the medicinal effectiveness of herbs. All of these books have their strengths. This one integrates all these kinds of information into a single, accessible, and practical book.

As an author, blogger, doctor, and researcher, I regularly search for information on herbs. I own dozens of herbal books and always grab a stack of them whenever I'm looking for information, because each book has its strength: information on growing herbs, therapeutic insights, or medicinal research. But I wanted a book that combines this information into a single, accessible, and practical book. *Be Your Own Herbalist* provides all the information you need to become a savvy home herbalist who can grow, use, and heal with these powerful medicines. With this book in hand, you can feel confident that you are using herbs safely and effectively. Growing and using natural medicines allows you to regain control over your own health and the health of your family, preventing and even reversing many serious health conditions. It is a step toward a life of self-sufficiency and independence.

Be Your Own Herbalist is loosely based on a series of articles I wrote for *Mother Earth Living* magazine from 2013 to the present, revised and expanded. It translates the most cutting-edge research on the therapeutic effectiveness of common herbs into accessible language illustrating just how therapeutic herbs can be while dispelling the myth that they are not as effective as other forms of medicine. It provides clear instructions for growing your own herbs in your garden, backyard, small farm, or even indoors or in pots on a balcony. It explains how to make your own salves, tinctures, herb-flavored honey, infused oils, compresses, and other herbal medicines. You'll find discussions of thirty-one of the most common and many of the most effective herbs that you can grow and use. Each chapter shares humorous or amusing information about the herb's historical uses, detailed growing instructions and harvesting guidelines, research that showcases the herb's effectiveness for various health conditions, and some recipes and suggestions for using the herb safely and effectively.

It is my mission in life to teach and empower people to become self-sufficient in growing their own food and natural medicines, and to use them to promote good health. How you opt to apply your knowledge of herbs is up to you. You may choose to use them for culinary purposes only, to enjoy more delicious and healthier foods. You may choose to use herbs alongside the pharmaceutical medicines you already use, to boost your overall health and strengthen your body. Or you may choose to use herbs as your primary system of medicine. Whatever choice you make, herbs can enrich and improve your health and life. Whether you simply want to dabble in using more fresh herbs for your cooking or whether you want to find greater food and medicine independence, you'll find the information you need to start or continue to use herbs in food and beverages, body-care products, and medicines. It also makes no difference whether you have a small apartment and can only grow medicines in pots on your windowsill, or whether you have a suburban patch of grass or a large acreage; you can still grow and use your own medicines. And even if you have no interest in growing herbs or making your own remedies, you can still use this book as a guide to help you navigate the waters of Mother Nature's medicine safely and for the benefit of your health and that of your family.

Before we begin, let me stress that you should always consult a physician if you are experiencing any symptoms of illness. If you are currently using other medications, research any possible herbal treatments carefully to avoid any adverse interactions. And, while this book is intended to give you the tools you need to incorporate herbal medicine into your health and life, it does not replace the expertise of a skilled herbalist, which can be invaluable in healing.

Now, allow me to take you on a miraculous journey that can help you reconnect to yourself and to the earth. If you have lost hope, allow me to light a candle of hope. There is always hope: it lies all around us in the form of herbal medicine.

2. Using Herbs: Know Your Infusions from Your Decoctions

Making your own herbal medicines and body-care products can save you money and improve your health, and it's much easier than you may think. If you already make herbal teas, making infused oils, tinctures, and salves can quickly become part of your repertoire too. In this chapter I share step-by-step instructions for making herbal remedies, as well as some essential therapeutic information to help you become your own home herbalist. Herbs can be used in many forms, including teas (infusions and decoctions), tinctures, wine infusions, vinegar infusions, glycerites, oil infusions, ointments and salves, lotions and creams, syrups, honeys, oxymels, poultices, and fomentations. Don't worry if this list sounds confusing; you'll soon discover how to harvest and prepare plants for different uses and learn everything you need to know to create home herbal medicines and body-care products.

Before you begin, always make sure that you are using the correct part of the plant, as some parts may be toxic if used internally.

Drying Herbs

One of the easiest ways to preserve an herb for future use is to dry it. The simplest way is to pick stems of the plant, tie them together in bunches no more than one inch in diameter, and hang them upside down in a dry, warm spot until all the plant matter becomes dry and brittle. You can also spread herbs out in a thin layer on a baking sheet and dry them in an oven at a low temperature (preferably 175°F or cooler) until the herbs dry. If you have a food dehydrator, set it to a low temperature setting (around 110°F) to dry herbs, spreading them out on trays. The amount of drying time varies significantly from herb to herb. Place the dried herbs in a glass jar with a tight seal, and store away from sunlight and moisture. Always make sure you label your herbs with the date of harvesting and the name (including the scientific name), to prevent possible confusion between similar herbs.

HOW LONG DO DRIED HERBS LAST?

Most leaves, flowers, and green parts of plants last for about one year after being dried. Roots, seeds, and bark may last for up to three years. Powdered or ground herbs tend to lose their medicinal and culinary value quickly and should be used within six months.

Tea Time

Making herbal tea may seem fairly straightforward, but if you want to reap the greatest medicinal value from the herbs you use, there's more to it than dunking a tea bag in hot water. There are two main forms of herbal tea: infusions and decoctions. Infusions are the commonly known form of herbal tea, in which herbs are literally infused in hot water, usually one heaping teaspoon of dried herb per cup of hot water for ten to twenty minutes. This is the ideal method for extracting the medicinal compounds in most berries, flowers, and leaves. You can also use fresh herbs, but because of their higher water content, you usually need to double the amount of herb matter per cup of water.

To extract the medicinal compounds from seeds, roots, or stems, you'll want to make a decoction, which involves boiling the herbs and allowing them to simmer for longer, about an hour, usually allowing one heaping teaspoon of dried herb per cup of water. Note that this method is less suitable for berries, flowers, and leaves because it tends to destroy many of the delicate medicinal compounds they contain. As with infusions, you can use fresh herbs, but you typically need to double the amount of herb matter used per cup of water.

What if you want to make a tea from some combination of roots, berries, seeds, stems, and leaves? Start by making a decoction with your chosen roots or seeds. Bring it to a boil, and then reduce to a simmer to continue brewing for an hour. Turn off the heat and add any berries, flowers, and leaves. Allow the herbal mixture to steep for an additional ten to twenty minutes. Now you've extracted the best medicinal compounds from all of the herbal components you're using.

Infused Oils: Massage and More

The infusion technique works to transfer the healing properties of herbs to oils as well as to water. Infused oils are excellent for massage or as a basis for balms and salves, which I discuss below.

Infused oils are simple to make. You can use any type of vegetable oil or carrier oil, other than petrochemical-based oils like baby oil or mineral oil; however, it is best to avoid oils that break down when exposed to heat, such as flaxseed oil. I prefer olive oil or sweet almond oil, which can be warmed to encourage the transfer of healing compounds from the herb matter to the oil. You can make many different types of infused oils, but two of the most common are St. John's wort and calendula oils.

St. John's wort oil, made from the flowers of the plant, is excellent for treating bruises, swellings, hemorrhoids, scars, and sprains.[1] Avoid sun exposure for a few hours after using this oil on your skin, as it can cause photosensitivity. Calendula oil, also made from the flowers of the plant, aids wound healing and alleviates various skin conditions.

There are two methods for making oil infusions: cold and warm. For flowers, which are delicate, it's best to use the cold method. This is also effective for the leaves of many plants. It involves adding fresh flowers or leaves to a jar and filling it with oil, such as sweet almond oil, apricot kernel oil, or extra-virgin olive oil. You'll want enough plant matter to ensure the medicinal value of the infused oil but not packed so tightly that the oil cannot penetrate the plant material. The plant material must be completely submerged in the oil to prevent mold from forming. Date and label the jar, and allow the infusion to rest for two weeks. You can shake the bottle periodically to encourage the infusion process. After two weeks, strain the herbs from the oil, squeezing out any remaining oil with clean hands. Cap and label the jar, and store away from light and heat.

The warm method involves placing the herbal matter in approximately the same volume of oil (or enough oil to cover) into a small Crock-Pot and allowing the mixture to "cook" on low heat for at least a few days, but preferably a week or two. Strain the herbs from the oil, squeezing out any remaining oil with clean hands. As with the cold method, pour the strained oil into a jar, cover with a lid, label, and store away from light and heat.

Infused oils can be used as is for massage or skin care or as a base for balms and salves.

Ointments, Balms, and Salves: Skin-Soothing Sensations

Salves and balms are basically herbal ointments made by thickening oil infusions with melted beeswax. Most health-food stores sell plain beeswax, which can be shaved with a potato peeler or grated with a cheese grater and then melted over low heat. Be sure to avoid other types of wax, since they are made of petroleum by-products.

Allow two tablespoons of shaved, melted beeswax to a cup of

infused oil after the herbal material has been strained off. Melt the beeswax over low heat to prevent overheating of the oil. Stir regularly. Remove from the heat as soon as the beeswax is melted and well incorporated into the oil. Pour into small, shallow jars, tins, or lip-balm containers. Let cool undisturbed to allow the ointment to set. Use for skin irritations and other skin conditions and for dry or chapped lips.

Creams and Lotions: Body Care with a Difference

If you're tired of all the chemicals and synthetic fragrances in store-bought creams and lotions, you might want to consider making your own. Most people think that making creams and body lotions is difficult, but it's actually quite easy. I frequently make my own and give them as gifts to friends and family members, who seem to love them.

I recommend that you keep an old blender, a small- to medium-sized glass bowl, and a spatula exclusively for making natural body-care products. Although it's safe to use your kitchen blender and food utensils, the beeswax used in natural creams can leave a residue on them.

As with salves and balms, you begin by melting beeswax into a plain or infused oil. Then you pour the oil-beeswax mixture into a blender and slowly pour in water or a strained herbal tea. As it blends, the oil mixture will thicken into a cream or lotion.

For the oil, you can either use an herbal infusion, such as peppermint, echinacea, or yarrow, or you can purchase essential oils, which are oils extracted from herbs. You can use both infusions and essential oils if you want to, but it is not necessary. Herbal teas usually create a milder-smelling lotion or cream than essential oils do, but both offer therapeutic value. Recipes for making creams and lotions appear throughout this book. With practice, you'll be able to vary the recipes to make products of different consistencies. For example, you might adjust a recipe depending on whether the cream is intended for oily or dry skin: the basic rule of thumb is less oil for oily skin, more for drier skin. But I encourage you to try the recipes in this book before you start experimenting, as you'll have a greater chance of success.

Syrups and Honeys: Sweet Solutions

Syrups and honeys are made by infusing herbs in sugar syrups or honey. I prefer to use honey because it is more natural than refined sugar and provides its own medicinal value, such as soothing the throat. Some herbs, like thyme and oregano, lend themselves well to cough syrups, since they have antiviral and antibacterial properties. Other herbs, like lavender, chive flowers, sage, and ginger, add uniquely delightful flavors to the already delicious taste of honey. You'll find a recipe for Honey-Thyme Cough Syrup on page 191.

Oxymels: Softening the Intensity of Herbs with Vinegar and Honey

Oxymels are simply blends of herbal honey with a little vinegar. They are often used for diluting the flavor of intensely strong herbs such as cayenne or garlic. To make an oxymel, measure one cup of vinegar into a pot. Add approximately two ounces of ground herb matter (except garlic, which should be added later). Bring the mixture to a boil, and let it simmer for fifteen minutes. Remove from the heat. If you're using fresh garlic, add it now. Let the mixture cool. Strain the herb material out of the vinegar, and add honey to the vinegar to taste. Simmer over low heat until it has the consistency of syrup. You can make an oxymel out of almost any herb you like — or even ones you don't like but whose medicinal benefits you would like to enjoy.

Tinctures: The Ultimate Herbal Medicine

Tinctures are alcohol extracts of either fresh or dried herbs. Sometimes just referred to as extracts, they are extremely effective at preserving the plant's active constituents. You can make a tincture from roots, leaves, seeds, stems, or flowers.

To make an herbal tincture, finely chop the fresh, clean herb you are using. You can also use dried herbs. Place the herb in a quart-sized glass jar. Fill the jar with as much plant matter as possible to ensure the medicinal value of your tincture, keeping in mind that you'll need enough alcohol to ensure the herbal matter is completely submerged. Top with vodka or pure grain alcohol, making sure all the plant matter is submerged in the alcohol to prevent mold growth. Date and label the jar, and allow the mixture to sit for two weeks, shaking daily to encourage extraction. After two weeks, strain the contents through a cheesecloth-lined sieve. After most of the liquid has gone through the sieve, pull up the corners of the cheesecloth, and, using clean hands, carefully wring out any remaining liquid. Store the herbal tincture in a jar, preferably away from heat or sunlight to preserve its healing properties. Tinctures usually keep for a few years. You can make an herbal tincture out of any medicinal or culinary herbs. A typical tincture dose is thirty drops three times daily unless otherwise specified.

While tinctures are excellent herbal medicines for most people, the alcohol base makes them unsuitable for people with certain health conditions, including pregnancy, liver disease, diabetes, or alcoholism. For most other circumstances, the small amount of alcohol is fine, but it's best to check with a qualified herbalist if you are uncertain.

Herbal Wines and Vinegars

Herbal wines and vinegars are made in the same way as tinctures, except that you use wine or vinegar in place of the vodka or grain alcohol. Obviously the taste will vary depending on the ingredients used. Not all herbs make great-tasting wine or vinegar, so select herbs you are familiar with. As with tinctures, you'll need to strain out the herbal matter through fine cheesecloth. Port, sherry, Madeira, mead, and even sparkling wine are all good candidates for making herbal wines.

To make herbal wine, simply grind the dried herb you're using to a coarse powder. Mix with the wine of your choice. Let it sit for fourteen days, shaking frequently. Strain it through cheesecloth, and pour into a sterilized bottle. Cap and store in a cool location. Herbal wine does not last as long as tinctures.

For herbal vinegars, use red or white wine vinegar or apple cider vinegar. To make herbal vinegars, follow the instructions for herbal wine, substituting the vinegar of your choice. Be sure to strain out all the herbal material before storing to prevent mold growth. The shelf life of herbal vinegars varies depending on the type of vinegar and herbs used, but in general it's best to use them within a month. Discard the vinegar if you notice mold formation.

Both herbal wines and vinegars can take some practice to perfect and are best attempted after you've gained some experience making some of the other herbal remedies.

Glycerites: Alcohol-Free Extracts

Glycerites are tinctures made with glycerin instead of alcohol and can be used instead of tinctures when needed. Glycerin is derived from the sweet-tasting components of fats and oils. It is available from most health-food stores and is typically made from coconut or vegetable oil. While glycerites taste sweet, they typically do not contain sugar. Glycerites tend to be inferior to alcohol extracts, infusions, decoctions, or oil infusions simply because fewer herb components are extracted with glycerin. I tend not to make them for this reason, but please keep me posted on your adventures making glycerites if you choose to try them.

Poultices: Herbs Got You Covered

A poultice is a paste made with herbs that is applied to the skin. It is typically applied while hot or warm, except when made with herbs that are naturally chemically hot, like chilis or ginger. To make a poultice, fill a natural-fiber cloth bag with powdered or chopped fresh herb matter. Tie it closed, and then place it into a bowl of hot water just long enough to soak and heat the herb. Remove it from the water, and apply to the affected area until the poultice has cooled and until you experience some relief. Reheat and reapply the poultice. It is best to use a fresh poultice every day.

Poultices are particularly effective in soothing aching or painful joints or muscles. Calendula helps bruises and damaged skin, echinacea boosts the immune system to help heal long-lasting wounds, and ginger is especially effective at reducing pain and throbbing.

The Fomentation Sensation

Fomentations are compresses made from herbal infusions or decoctions. A cloth soaked in an herbal tea is applied to an affected area. A fomentation can be used hot or cold, depending on the application. Cold fomentations work well on areas that are inflamed, while hot fomentations work well to relieve the pain of sore muscles. A cold fomentation can be used on an injured joint or headache, while a hot fomentation relieves tightness and soreness in muscles. You may already be familiar with using black tea compresses to treat conjunctivitis (pinkeye).

It may feel a bit overwhelming to try to remember all of these terms and how to make these different remedies. But you can simply refer back to this chapter whenever you need some herbal relief. With a little effort, you'll be a pro in no time.

Ethical Wildcrafting and Herbal Medicine Use

We are all stewards of the planet on which we live, and we share the responsibility to care for it. As the Haudenosaunee Native American Ely Parker once said, "We are connected to a community, but a community that transcends time."[2] Caring for our global community means respecting and nurturing the herbs and plants that grow upon the earth. While you may plan to grow many of your own medicinal plants, here are some ethical guidelines for gathering wild plants:

1. Learn which species of herbs are endangered (a list that can vary over time), and avoid their use. Wild ginseng and goldenseal have been harvested nearly to the point of extinction, and

while both are valuable herbs, I have not included them among the herb profiles because I do not wish to contribute to further harvesting of these endangered plant species.

2. Recognize that every time we remove a plant from its growing place, we need to leave others to ensure the survival of the species. Obviously, with plants that are highly prolific, such as dandelion, this is not as much of a concern as it is with endangered species. But few herbs can match dandelion's inherent ability to grow and spread; most herbs require us to be cautious and considerate when harvesting them.

3. If you need only the leaves or flower of the plant, then harvest only those parts. This may seem obvious, but some people unthinkingly uproot a plant, killing it unnecessarily.

4. Do not harvest too many different types of plants in a single day unless you are certain that you will have the time and energy to process them. It's important not to waste these precious plants.

5. Avoid wildcrafting on private property unless you have received the permission of the owner.

6. Respect the plants' habitat as well as individual plants. Avoid harvesting herbs in vulnerable, compromised, damaged, or at-risk areas in which the removal of plants could adversely affect other species or the sustainability of that ecosystem. If you walk your dog or other animal while harvesting, keep it leashed and avoid habitats where the animal may cause harm, such as nesting areas for birds.

7. Avoid harvesting in any national park areas, which is illegal.

8. For your own safety, avoid harvesting plants near roadsides, highways, brownfields, or other polluted areas, as environmental toxins can become concentrated in the plants harvested there.

Now let's begin our exploration of the exciting world of herbal medicines.

PART 2

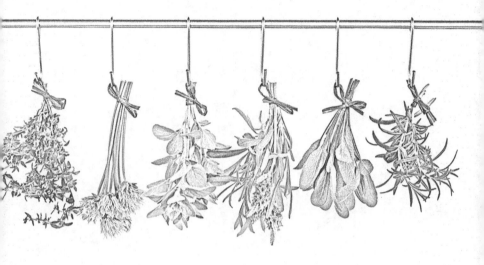

Discovering Nature's
Herbal Wonders

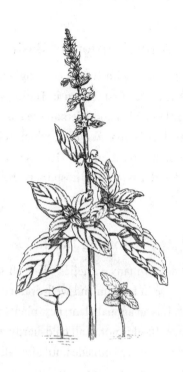

3. Basil

Ocimum basilicum

I still remember the first time I tasted basil — and the Italian restaurant that served up this little bit of heaven. It transformed a plain tomato salad into an extraordinary taste sensation. Basil accompanies tomatoes beautifully both in the garden and on the plate, and it's the star in traditional pesto. But this aromatic and delicious plant has much more to offer than just its striking aroma and flavor.

A Brief History of Basil

Most people associate basil with Italian cooking, so it may come as a surprise to learn that it was first grown in India, Asia, and Africa. It plays a prominent role in Thai and Vietnamese cuisine. Its name originates from the Greek adjective *basilikon*, which refers to a coin with the emperor's head on it. To the ancient Greeks it was a sacred herb. In India basil is considered a symbol of hospitality. In Italy it symbolizes love.

Growing Basil

Although basil comes in many varieties, they all generally need the same care. Basils thrive in full sun and well-drained soil enriched with compost or manure. It is an annual plant; new plants can be started from seed or from cuttings. Basil is not at all cold-hardy, so plants should be started indoors and not planted outside until after all signs of frost have passed. In cool climates, it grows better indoors, as long as it gets plenty of light. Although it loves heat, basil needs plenty of water.

Basil plants grow one to two feet tall. The taste differs depending on the variety, with flavor notes ranging from cinnamon and clove to lemon or lime. Leaf color also varies from bright green to dark purple by variety. Try classic, deep green Genovese for classic pesto; purple Red Rubin for its spice; and light-green lemon basil for its incredible aroma. Pinch off the edible flower heads regularly (add them to salads or stir-fries) to encourage the plant to put its energy into growing thick foliage; otherwise the plants may become spindly.

Harvesting Basil

Although its flavor is strong, basil is versatile in the kitchen. Try its leaves in soups, salads, stews, pesto, pasta, and tomato sauce; alongside tomatoes, peppers, and eggplant; and in curries made with coconut milk. It is best to add the fresh leaves just before serving, as they lose their robust flavor and aroma after heating. Harvest the leaves whenever the plant looks as if it can spare a few, but resist the temptation to overharvest; leave at least a few leaves to ensure that the plant survives. The leaves bruise easily, so handle them carefully.

Most basils are prolific producers. To preserve basil, most cooks prefer freezing, as dried basil tastes very different from fresh and much less robust. It's easy to capture the fresh flavor of basil by puréeing the leaves in a food processor in a base of water or olive oil (not both), pouring the mixture into ice-cube trays, and freezing. Once frozen, bag the cubes and add them as desired to cooked soups, stews, and sauces. For use in teas, which produce a more potent extract, dried basil leaves may be preferable.

Once the plant is mature, you can dry leaves on the stem by cutting a stalk at the base of the plant and hanging it upside down for a few days or until the leaves are dry. Over a clean sheet, collect the dried leaves, and use as desired for tea or in cooking.

Using Basil

Infection Fighter

Basil has been shown to have excellent anti-infectious qualities. Research in the journal *Molecules* found that the natural volatile oils in basil inhibited multiple drug-resistant strains of *E. coli* bacteria.[1] (*E. coli*, which can be contracted from contaminated food, causes cramps, diarrhea, and vomiting.) In a preliminary study published in *BMC Complementary and Alternative Medicine*, scientists demonstrated that an extract of basil seeds was effective in the laboratory against tuberculosis-causing bacteria.[2]

Pain Reliever

Eugenol, one of the beneficial compounds in basil, has been studied extensively for its ability to fight pain by suppressing the body's production of the enzyme cyclooxygenase (COX) — a mechanism similar to but more effective than the one used by aspirin and ibuprofen, which merely prevents binding to this enzyme to alleviate pain. To try it at home, brew basil tea by adding a teaspoon of dried basil or a tablespoon of fresh basil leaves to a cup of boiled water and letting it steep for ten minutes. Strain and drink.

Breath Freshener

Basil freshens breath. Simply chew on a fresh basil leaf or drink a cup of basil tea.

Blood Pressure Balancer

According to the research of the renowned botanist James Duke, basil contains six natural compounds that reduce high blood pressure, making it a great regular dietary addition for anyone suffering from the condition.[3]

Cancer Remedy

Exciting new research published in the journal *Molecular Medicine Reports* found that an extract of basil halted ovarian cancer cell growth. Eating basil on a regular basis may help stave off cancer.[4]

Wart Remover

Basil's antiviral compounds go to work when the crushed leaves are applied to warts. Crush a fresh leaf or two, place on the wart, and cover with a bandage. Change the compress daily for five to seven days. Repeat the process if necessary.

RECIPES

Basil Butter

This recipe combines the health benefits of coconut oil (which is effective against infections) and flaxseed oil (a natural anti-inflammatory) with the beneficial properties of basil. Serve this soft spread on warm bread, or add to vegetables after cooking to maximize the basil flavor and avoid destroying the beneficial omega-3 fatty acids found in flaxseed oil. It's simple to make and keeps well in the fridge. It adds a fresh, gourmet flavor to almost any dish.

Makes about 1 cup.

½ cup organic extra-virgin coconut oil
½ cup organic cold-pressed flaxseed oil
Large handful of fresh basil leaves, chopped

In a small saucepan over low heat, melt the coconut oil. Immediately remove from the heat and add the flaxseed oil, stirring until well mixed. Stir in the basil. Pour into a glass container with a lid, cover, and refrigerate until firm. Store in an airtight container in the refrigerator for up to six months.

Pineapple-Basil Quinoa

The combination of pineapple and basil gives this whole-grain side dish a unique flavor. Quinoa only takes about 15 minutes to cook, making it the ultimate protein-, fiber-, and nutrient-rich fast food.

Serves 4.

1 cup quinoa, rinsed to reduce bitterness
1½ cups water
2 tablespoons coconut oil, divided
Large handful of fresh basil leaves, chopped
¾ cup finely diced fresh pineapple
½ teaspoon sea salt

Combine the quinoa, water, and 1 tablespoon of coconut oil in a medium pot. Bring to a boil.

Cover, reduce the heat to low, and simmer for 15 to 20 minutes, or until the water is absorbed.

In a mixing bowl, toss together the cooked quinoa with the remaining coconut oil, basil, pineapple, and salt until combined. Serve immediately.

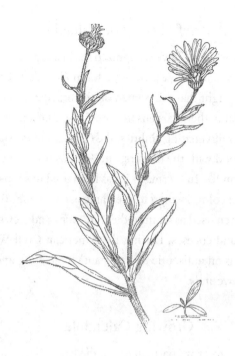

4. Calendula

Calendula officinalis

Calendula is best known for its beautiful flowers. Gardeners more often refer to it as marigold or pot marigold. While this natural beauty certainly adds a sunny yellow or orange burst of color to gardens and flowering baskets, it also offers much more for our health and well-being. It has been used medicinally since the twelfth century for wounds, insect bites, fungal conditions, and many other skin conditions. Increasing amounts of research document the many medicinal properties of calendula.

A Brief History of Calendula

Many cultures worldwide have recognized the healing benefits of calendula. The plant's name comes from the Latin *kalends*, because the ancient Romans thought that it bloomed on the first day of every month. They cultivated it in their gardens to spread joy. The ancient Egyptians revered it for its rejuvenating abilities, the Greeks and Persians flavored and garnished food with the flowers, and Hindus use it to decorate the altars in their temples. In Germany it has been used in soups and broths to add flavor and color, leading to the name *pot marigold*. Elsewhere in Europe, it has been used as an ingredient in soups and stews and to add color to butter and cheeses. During the American Civil War, doctors used calendula as an antiseptic and to staunch bleeding and speed the healing of open wounds.[1]

Growing Calendula

Calendula is easy to grow, particularly in the late spring, early summer, and late autumn, since it prefers cooler weather. It grows best in full sun or partially shady areas or in containers. Although it is an annual, it readily self-seeds, making it a plant you can enjoy year after year. It usually grows to between one and two feet tall and flowers from late spring until mid-fall, making it a lovely addition to your garden throughout the growing season. Sow the seeds about a week before the last frost. In a week or two you'll notice the greenery poking its head above the earth. If flower production slows at the height of summer, simply cut the plants back to about half of their original size to encourage blooming. Remove the dead flowers (a practice known as "deadheading") to boost the production of new flowers.

Harvesting Calendula

The flowers are primarily used either as an addition to salads or in making salves, ointments, and tinctures to apply topically. Like saffron, the dried flowers add a yellow hue to dishes. The leaves can also be used in soups and salads or as a garnish. Both the flowers and the leaves can be dried for longer storage.

Using Calendula

If you are using the plant internally or topically, be sure you are using the *Calendula officinalis* variety and not another type of calendula, since some are not suitable for these purposes. Avoid internal use during pregnancy. Avoid use of this herb if you suffer from hay fever or if you experience any allergic reaction.

Bug Bite Reliever

If you've been bitten by a mosquito or flea, salves made with calendula can stop the itching.

Bunion Aid

Calendula has been traditionally recommended for relieving the pain and inflammation of bunions. Apply a calendula salve or tincture directly to the bunion two or three times daily for a week to determine whether it will help you.

Cancer Treatment Reliever

In a study published in the *Journal of the Advanced Practitioner in Oncology* of women who received radiotherapy for breast cancer, calendula ointment was more effective than the drug used for treating the painful skin conditions caused by the radiation treatment.[2]

Gingivitis Fighter

Calendula's antibacterial and immune system–stimulating properties make it helpful in the treatment of gingivitis. This is a mild and common form of gum disease that manifests as irritation, swelling, and inflammation of the gums. A study published in the *Journal of the Indian Society of Periodontology* assessed the traditional use of calendula mouthwash in the treatment of gingivitis. Over six months, one group of study participants used a mouthwash made from calendula tincture and water, while the second group used a placebo mouthwash. The researchers found a significant reduction in dental plaque, gingivitis, and gum bleeding in the group that used the calendula mouthwash.[3]

Skin Healer

Researchers at the Medical Biotechnology School of Medicine at Flinders University in Australia assessed the purported antioxidant and therefore skin-healing properties of calendula. In a study published in *Phytotherapy Research*, they found that a calendula extract worked on human skin cells as an antioxidant and boosted healing.[4] What's more, the Commission E, the German government's expert committee on medicinal herbs, endorses calendula for reducing inflammation and promoting healing.[5]

Wound Healer Extraordinaire

Calendula has commonly been used in the form of a salve, ointment, or tincture to promote wound healing. In another study published in *Phytotherapy Research*, researchers assessed the effectiveness of this traditional remedy in tincture form. They found that calendula increased the rate of wound healing by increasing the number of the body's immune system cells that destroy harmful invaders like bacteria, viruses, and fungi.[6]

RECISES

Calendula Ointment or Salve

While calendula ointments or salves are readily available in most health-food stores, they are also easy to make at home. Keep some on hand to treat rashes, burns, wounds, and other skin conditions.

Makes approximately 1 cup.

¼ cup dried calendula petals or flower heads
½ cup extra-virgin olive oil
⅛ cup grated beeswax

In a small pot, heat the calendula and oil on low until the oil is warm but not hot (approximately 10 minutes). Cover and let the mixture sit for at least one hour. Slowly pour the oil mixture through a cheesecloth-lined sieve into a glass or ceramic dish or bowl. Pour the strained olive oil back into the pot, add the beeswax, and heat on low, stirring gently until the beeswax is melted. Again, the oil should be warm but not hot. Pour the mixture into clean glass jars, leaving it undisturbed and uncovered until completely cooled. Cover and label the jars. The ointment should last at least one year if stored in the refrigerator. Use topically on skin conditions and wounds.

Calendula Mouthwash

This mouthwash is based on the one used in the gingivitis study cited above. Make it fresh on a weekly basis.
    Makes ½ cup.

    1 ounce calendula tincture
    3 ounces distilled water

Mix the tincture with the water. Use the mouthwash at least once a day for best results.

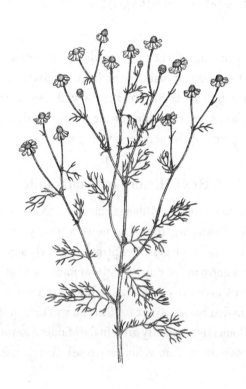

5. Chamomile

Chamaemelum nobile, Matricaria chamomilla,
Matricaria recutita

Twenty-two years ago I opened a health-food store. Things were quite different in the field of herbalism back then. Few of my clients took any medications; today, it's common for people to come in with grocery bags holding all their pharmaceutical drugs. Few people gave herbs a second thought, but now herbal medicine is increasingly being recognized as a safe and effective form of treatment. Even then, however, people understood that chamomile, a small plant with tiny flowers, was a potent medicine. Ironically, while there is more research than ever showcasing chamomile's medicinal benefits, many people seem to have forgotten this valuable herb. I hope that after you read the exciting information about chamomile, you will restore it to its rightful place in your home and natural medicine cabinet, and maybe even add a container or patch of chamomile to your garden.

A Brief History of Chamomile

Chamomile is proof that good things come in small packages. When it blooms, it showcases tiny, daisy-like flowers with yellow centers and white petals, and feathery leaves. The plant has a lovely apple-like scent. It grows wild in some parts of Europe and was introduced to North America by early settlers or explorers. Although we don't know exactly when chamomile was first harvested as a medicine, it was used in ancient Egypt, Greece, and Rome. Its popularity grew in the Middle Ages as a remedy for health concerns ranging from asthma to nausea, skin diseases, and fevers.

Growing Chamomile

There are different types of chamomile, including German, Roman, Hungarian, and wild chamomile. The German type (*Matricaria chamomilla* or *Matricaria recutita*) and the Roman (*Chamaemelum nobile*) are the most common. German chamomile is an annual plant that grows as tall as three feet and can produce quite large flowers, whereas Roman chamomile is a perennial plant that grows closer to the ground and has smaller flowers. Both can be grown from seeds or seedlings indoors or outside, in pots or directly in your garden.

Harvesting Chamomile

Chamomile's healing properties are derived from the flowers, which can be used fresh or dried and kept in a jar. To dry the flowers, hang the cut stems, with flowers intact, upside down in bunches, and remove and store the flowers when completely dry. It is best to avoid using chamomile if you are allergic to ragweed. Also, the drug warfarin (Coumadin) has been found to interact with chamomile. Other blood thinners may also interact with chamomile, so it is best not to use chamomile if you are taking these drugs.

Using Chamomile

Since the flowers are the part of the plant with the most beneficial properties, they are best made into water or oil infusions, dried and added to baths or body-care products, or made into tinctures. Roman or German chamomile can be prepared in the same way. It is easy to make an infusion with chamomile that can be used daily to reap its healing properties. The infusion can be stored in the refrigerator for up to three days.

Skin Treatment and Stomach Cramp Solution

Germany's Commission E approved German chamomile as a treatment of the skin to reduce swelling and fight bacteria, as well as a tea or supplement to alleviate stomach cramps.[1]

Dental Antimicrobial

Researchers assessed the antimicrobial activity of an extract of German chamomile against the fungus *Candida albicans* and the bacterium *Enterococcus faecalis*. *C. albicans* is a common fungal condition (sometimes, albeit less accurately, referred to as a yeast infection), and *E. faecalis* is an antibiotic-resistant and often life-threatening infection that sometimes inhabits root-canal-treated teeth. The *Indian Journal of Dentistry* published an assessment of a high-potency extract of chamomile against these microbes and found that it helped kill both.[2] This study could help explain German chamomile's reputation for healing dental abscesses and gum inflammation.

Mouthwash for Mouth Ulcerations

A study in the *Journal of Clinical and Experimental Dentistry* found that a mouthwash made of German chamomile was effective at treating mouth ulcerations and the associated pain and did so without any side effects.[3]

Skin Healer

Chamomile is often used by herbalists in the treatment of skin conditions like chicken pox rash, diaper rash, eczema, and psoriasis. For these purposes it is usually added to a bath or applied to the skin as an infusion or alcohol extract. Keep in mind, however, that the alcohol in extracts can be drying to the skin.

Liver Protector

In a new animal study published in the medical journal *General Physiology and Biophysics*, researchers found that a decoction of German chamomile protected the livers of animals against the damaging effects of alcohol, suggesting the potential for liver protection for humans as well.[4] Further research is needed to study this possible application, but considering that chamomile has proven itself a valuable healer with almost no side effects, it may be worth a try.

Antioxidant Power

In a study published in the *Journal of Chromatography A*, researchers compared the antioxidant power of German chamomile to that of feverfew and calendula and found that chamomile had the highest antioxidant potency, making it helpful in mitigating the free-radical damage to cells that is linked to aging and most diseases.[5]

Anti-inflammatory

A study published in the *Journal of Natural Products* assessed the purported anti-inflammatory properties of Roman chamomile. Researchers found that it contains at least one anti-inflammatory compound and can even be beneficial in treating metabolic syndrome, a group of symptoms that includes high blood sugar, cholesterol, and homocysteine levels.[6] In addition to these three markers, metabolic syndrome is characterized by abdominal fat and is often a precursor of other health conditions. Homocysteine is a marker of inflammation and can increase the risk of over fifty diseases, so reducing these substances can have significant health benefits.

Tumor Fighter

Additional research in the journal *Food Chemistry* found that Roman chamomile had both antioxidant and antitumor properties. It also found that an infusion of chamomile had significantly greater antioxidant and antitumor effects than a decoction or extract.[7] This research reinforces the advice that making an infusion or herbal tea yields the greatest therapeutic benefits of using herb flowers.

RECIPE

Soothing Chamomile Cream

This silky cream soothes inflammation as it glides across the skin. It is simple to make and doesn't require a lot of ingredients. Because there are no chemical preservatives used, it is a good idea to store this cream in the refrigerator.

Makes about 2 cups.

1 cup water
2 teaspoons dried chamomile flowers (or 4 teaspoons fresh Roman chamomile flowers)
¾ cup sweet almond or apricot kernel oil (available in most health-food stores)
2 tablespoons shaved beeswax

Boil the water and pour it over the chamomile flowers. Cover the mixture and let it brew for 10 to 20 minutes. Strain out the flowers, reserving the chamomile-infused water. Set aside.

Pour the oil into a Pyrex measuring cup, and add the shaved beeswax. Set the measuring cup in a saucepan of water that reaches about halfway up the side of the measuring cup. Heat the mixture until the beeswax dissolves, and then remove the measuring cup from the heat immediately. Allow it to cool for a minute or two, but not longer, as the beeswax will begin to harden.

Pour the chamomile-infused water into a blender, cover, and begin blending it on high speed. With the blender running, slowly pour the beeswax mixture through the hole in the blender lid. The mixture will begin to thicken after about three-quarters of the beeswax mixture has been incorporated.

Once all the beeswax has been blended, immediately pour the lotion into one 16-ounce glass jar or two 8-ounce glass jars. Use a spatula to remove any remaining lotion from the blender.

The lotion lasts about 3 months in the fridge.

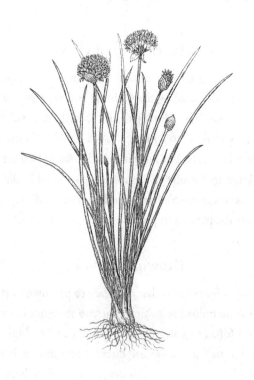

6. Chives

Allium schoenoprasum

Most people think of chives as a garnish atop a soup, stew, or salad. But chives warrant consideration as both a dietary and medicinal staple, particularly as we deal with increasingly virulent infections and rapidly rising rates of cancer. Chives have been found to be effective against serious bacterial infections as well as in preventing and treating cancer. This beautiful perennial herb is a great addition to almost any savory meal and a lovely enhancement to any garden.

A Brief History of Chives

Chives have been in use for over five thousand years. Native to Asia, chives were originally used by the Chinese and now are a part of many cuisines throughout Asia, Europe, and North America.[1] Colonists brought chives with them to America.[2] As a member of the allium family, chives are relatives of both garlic and onions.[3] Over a century ago, chives were used in fortune-telling. A person would take a bunch of chive stalks, toss them onto a bare wooden table, and the fortune-teller would interpret the pattern to predict the client's future.[4]

Growing Chives

Chives are grown from bulbs that continue to produce every year with minimal care. The bulbs are so tiny that you may not even know they are there. The foliage grows about eighteen inches high in clusters, like grass, except that the stalks are circular and hollow inside. Chives thrive in most climates. When in bloom, they produce beautiful pink to lavender flowers, making them a great addition to decorative and edible gardens alike. Chives prefer well-drained and thoroughly weeded soil, and they need adequate space. Plant about six bulbs in a cluster about eight inches from the nearest plants or other chive clusters. Every few years, divide the chive bulbs and move some of them to a new location. They require minimal water. The easiest way to tell when chives need watering is to inspect the tips of the leaves. If they look a bit dry, it's time to water the plant. Avoid any heavy applications of nitrogen fertilizers.[5] In the garden, chives help to repel some insects and mildew.[6] They are also easy to grow indoors or outdoors in pots.

Harvesting Chives

Using scissors, snip the outer leaves of chives as needed about two inches above the base of the plant. After the plant has flowered, snip the flowering stems back to about two inches as well. To dry chives, cut off sprigs about two inches above the soil, wash, lay out on a baking sheet, and dry in a 175°F (if possible) or 200°F oven for an hour or two or until completely dry. Once they are dry, store them whole or cut into small pieces in an airtight container for up to a year. Fresh chive flowers are also edible (just ask the deer in my area) and are delicious atop a mixed green salad or soup. The fresh or dried leaves are a delicious addition to potato and fish dishes. They are a traditional addition to the Russian and Polish soft cheese known as tvorog, but they can also be used with any soft dairy or vegan cheese.[7] Chives are also a delicious addition to gravies and sauces.

Using Chives

Antibacterial Wonder

In a study published in the medical journal *Molecules*, French scientists found that chives demonstrated antibacterial action against the five strains of bacteria they tested, including *Staphylococcus*, *Listeria*, *Salmonella*, *Campylobacter*, and *E. coli*. They also found that chives were most effective against these bacteria when used in their natural, raw state and that they lost effectiveness when heated.[8]

Cancer-Prevention Powerhouse

Exciting new research published in the medical journal *Cancer Prevention Research* found that chives have potent cancer-prevention properties, particularly against gastrointestinal cancers. The researchers at the National Cancer Institute and the U.S. Department of Agriculture believe that the sulfur compounds naturally present in chives are likely responsible for the herb's impressive anticancer effects.[9]

Cancer Fighter

Not only do chives help prevent cancer, but the herb has also been found to stop existing cancer cells from proliferating, thereby halting or slowing the spread of cancer. While most studies have examined the use of chive leaves, in a study published in the medical journal *Molecules*, researchers assessed the anticancer properties of chive flowers. According to their findings, not only are chive flowers pretty to look at, but they are also a potent anticancer medicine.[10]

Sore Throat Aid

Scientists at the Iuliu Hatieganu University of Medicine and Pharmacy in Romania assessed the traditional use of chives to relieve sore throats. Their findings, published in the *Journal of Physiology and Pharmacology*, indicate that an alcohol extract of chives is an effective sore-throat remedy, largely because of the herb's potent anti-inflammatory properties.[11]

RECIPE

Dairy-Free Soft Cheese with Chives

This is my favorite probiotic-rich, dairy-free cheese. It is super-creamy and sliceable and even melts well, although heating it will destroy the beneficial cultures. The cheese can be enjoyed on its own or with a drizzle of balsamic vinegar, fresh fruit, crackers, or fresh bread.

Makes 1 medium-sized block of cheese.

1 cup raw unsalted cashews
1 cup water, preferably filtered or unchlorinated
1 probiotic capsule or ½ teaspoon probiotic powder
⅓ cup coconut oil, melted but not hot
1 tablespoon dark miso
⅓ teaspoon sea salt
2 tablespoons chopped fresh or dried chives

Soak the cashews in the water for 8 hours or overnight. Strain the cashews, reserving the soaking water. Blend the cashews and ½ cup of the soaking water together in a blender or with an immersion blender until smooth. Pour the mixture into a glass or ceramic bowl. Empty the contents of the probiotic capsule or add the probiotic powder to the mixture; stir until well blended. Cover with a cloth, and allow the cheese to ferment for 8 to 12 hours, according to taste. Shorter fermentation times create a milder cheese; longer times develop a stronger cheese flavor.

Blend together the cashew mixture, coconut oil, miso, and salt. Once they are blended, gently stir in the chives. Pour the cheese into a small glass bowl lined with cheesecloth, stirring to remove air pockets. Allow it to chill in the refrigerator until firm, at least two hours. Remove the cheese from the bowl, and serve immediately or store in an airtight container in the fridge.

The cheese will typically keep for one month when refrigerated.

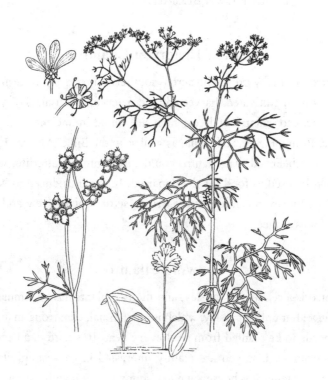

7. Cilantro

Coriandrum sativum

Is there any herb more versatile and yet more underrated than cilantro? Often excluded from the herb section of gardens, this plant deserves a second look. It is a key ingredient in cuisines from almost every continent, and it gives you two delicious yet entirely distinct flavors: one from the leaves and one from the dried seed. While the entire plant is often referred to as coriander, *cilantro* refers to the leaves and stalks, and *coriander* to the seeds.

A Brief History of Cilantro

Cilantro originally grew wild across southern Europe and eastern Asia and has been cultivated, harvested, and eaten for thousands of years. References to cilantro and coriander are found in ancient texts from China, Rome, Egypt, and India, as well as in the Bible. Ancient Egyptians even believed that cilantro could travel into the afterlife, where it could be used as food for the departed. It was introduced to North America by seventeenth-century British settlers, who grew and harvested it as a spice.

Growing Cilantro

Cilantro is a relative of parsley, and the two plants have a similar appearance; but unlike parsley, which is a perennial, cilantro is an annual and needs to be planted from seed every year. It is hardy and easy to grow from seed. If you are mainly interested in harvesting cilantro leaves and stems, it is best grown in a sunny location with partial shade to encourage foliage growth; however, if you want to grow it for seeds, plant it in a location with full sun. Sow the seeds about half an inch deep and spaced a few inches apart. For a continuous supply, sow additional seeds every two weeks. Cilantro can also be grown indoors in containers. It needs moderate amounts of water and minimal organic fertilizer.

Harvesting Cilantro

All parts of the plant, including the root, are edible, but most recipes call for either the leaves or the seeds. Once the cilantro produces leaves (usually by early summer), you can harvest up to one-third of the plant's leaves. As the plant grows larger, you can cut whole stems. The stems have the same flavor as the leaves and can be used the same way. Simply chop them finely, and add to your favorite dish.

If you want coriander seeds, you'll need to wait until the plant sends up a long flower stalk, blooms, and goes to seed, which usually happens by late summer. I find it easiest to harvest the seeds by waiting until they turn brown on the plant, cutting the plant from the base, and shaking it upside down over a wide bowl to catch the falling seeds.

Store the seeds in an airtight jar, and use them in your favorite soups, stews, salad dressings, and curries. You can sauté them whole in a small amount of oil to soften them and bring out the flavor before adding other ingredients, or grind them to a fine powder and add as desired to your recipe.

Cilantro is truly an international herb. Fans of Mexican and Tex-Mex food will be familiar with the generous use of cilantro leaves in many dishes, including salsa and guacamole. Indian cuisine is chock-full of both the leaves and the seeds in curry dishes. You'll also find cilantro in many Thai dishes and authentic Chinese foods.

Using Cilantro

Blood Sugar Balancer

Cilantro was traditionally used in parts of Europe and North Africa to combat diabetes. In 2011, a team of Moroccan scientists decided to test its efficacy in an animal study. They found that when cilantro was added to the diets of rats, it not only improved or normalized many metabolic symptoms of diabetes but also improved symptoms linked to cardiovascular disease.[1]

Cholesterol Normalizer

One of the reasons that cilantro may be effective against cardio-vascular disease is that it helps keep arteries free of fatty deposits and plaque that build up when low-density lipoprotein (LDL) cholesterol molecules are oxidized by free radicals. LDL cholesterol is known as the "bad" cholesterol. Free radicals — chemical compounds that are unstable because they are missing an electron — wreak havoc in the body as they try to steal electrons from molecules in healthy cells (often damaging the DNA of these cells in the process). They are linked to accelerated aging and disease. Cilantro is high in the flavonoid quercetin, which slows the oxidation of LDL cholesterol and potentially protects artery walls from damage as well.[2] Flavonoids are a group of highly medicinal compounds found in certain plant-based foods.

Inflammation Reducer

Cilantro has long been used in Ayurvedic medicine to combat inflammation. Scientists at the All-India Institute of Medical Sciences in New Delhi put tradition to the test in 2010 by evaluating the effectiveness of extracts of *Coriandrum sativum* against arthritis. They found that the extract helped to reduce joint inflammation in the test animals.[3]

---

10 SIMPLE WAYS TO USE CILANTRO

Toss freshly chopped leaves into:

Salsa
Guacamole
Stir-fries
Stews
Curries
Pesto, in place of basil
Chili
Salad
Asian noodle dishes like pad thai
Olives, with a little lemon zest

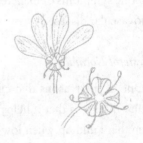

RECIPES

Pink Salad with Superbly Cilantro Dressing

This delicious salad takes less than ten minutes to make, including the homemade dressing.

Serves 2 to 4.

Dressing
- ¼ cup cold-pressed flaxseed oil
- ½ cup extra-virgin olive oil
- ⅓ cup freshly squeezed lemon juice
- Pinch of unrefined sea salt
- Large handful of fresh cilantro
- Handful of fresh parsley (optional)
- 1 clove garlic
- 2 teaspoons unpasteurized honey

Salad
- 2 cups leafy greens of your choice (spring mix, romaine lettuce, butter lettuce, etc.)
- Half a carrot, grated
- 1 small beet, grated
- Handful of raw, unsalted pumpkin seeds

Blend all the dressing ingredients together in a blender, or use an immersion blender to blend them in a jar. Blend until smooth. You won't need all the dressing for this salad. Store the remaining dressing in a closed jar in the refrigerator.

Assemble the leafy greens, carrot, and beet on a large plate or bowl. Top with the dressing and the pumpkin seeds.

Super-Simple and Delicious Black Bean Chili

This yummy black bean chili is perfect for a cold autumn or winter evening, but it's so good that you'll probably want to enjoy it in every season. It's simple to make. I put the dried beans in a slow cooker in the morning and then simply add the remaining ingredients an hour or so before dinnertime. If you don't have time to cook dried beans (which usually takes 2 to 4 hours on high, depending on your slow cooker), substitute 4 cups of canned beans, drained and rinsed. Cook for at least 30 minutes, or longer if you prefer, to allow the flavors to develop. If you prefer kidney beans, feel free to substitute them for the black beans. The quinoa is optional, but it adds even more protein to this already protein-rich vegan dinner. Cumin adds amazing flavor to the chili. With 15 grams of fiber per cup of black beans (a typical amount in a serving of chili), this dish also helps keep you regular.

Serves 6.

1½ cups dried black beans
9 cups water, divided
2 tablespoons extra-virgin olive oil
2 onions, chopped
3 carrots, chopped
2 red bell peppers, chopped
1 stalk celery, chopped
One 24-ounce jar tomato sauce
1 cup quinoa (optional), rinsed to reduce bitterness
2 teaspoons ground cumin
1 teaspoon unrefined sea salt
½ teaspoon chili powder
Large handful of fresh cilantro leaves and stems, chopped
Guacamole or slices of avocado for garnish (optional)

In a medium to large slow cooker, combine the beans and 6 cups of the water. Cover and cook on low for 6 to 8 hours or on high for 3 to 4 hours. Drain and rinse. Return the beans to the slow cooker.

In a large skillet, heat the oil over medium-low heat, making sure it never smokes. Sauté the onions for 5 minutes. Add the carrots, peppers, and celery; sauté the vegetables for 10 minutes, or until the onions are lightly browned. Transfer the vegetables to the slow cooker.

Add the tomato sauce, quinoa (if you're using it), cumin, salt, chili powder, cilantro, and remaining water to the slow cooker. Cover and cook on a low setting for 1 to 1½ hours, or until the quinoa is tender.

Garnish each bowl with a dollop of guacamole or a few slices of avocado if desired.

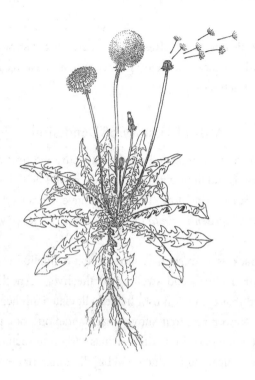

8. Dandelion

Taraxacum officinale

The dandelion is an herb in serious need of an image makeover. Cursed by many gardeners and those in quest of perfect lawns, dandelion is frequently viewed as a pest plant. If you walk past my home, you'll know it from the dandelions that grow rampant on the front lawn. While my neighbors continue to douse the yellow flowers with harmful pesticides, I prefer to let the resilient and prevalent flowers grow. That's because, in addition to dandelion's excellent nutritional benefits, it has scientifically proven medicinal properties and an extensive history of use. Research is increasingly showing its benefits for fighting cancer, preventing osteoporosis, treating Alzheimer's disease, and much more.

A Brief History of Dandelion

An Arab doctor first recorded dandelion's curative properties in the tenth century. Dandelion was once called "piddle bed" because of its ability to increase urine flow. The French have a less tactful name for the plant as well: *pissenlit. En lit* means "in bed." I'll leave you to figure out the rest.

As far back as 1880, studies showed that dandelion is an effective treatment for hepatitis and swelling of the liver.[1] Another German study proved that dandelion root helped alleviate jaundice and reduce gallstones.[2] Newer research shows that dandelion root protects the liver against some harmful toxins, such as carbon tetrachloride, which is used in some cleaning products and building materials.[3]

Growing Dandelion

I probably don't have to give you any advice on how to grow dandelion, other than to avoid using pesticides and to cut your grass less often. By cutting your grass less frequently, you'll increase the likelihood that the yellow dandelion flowers will go to seed (forming the familiar puffball heads). When that happens, the wind disperses the seeds and helps ensure that more dandelion plants grow in your yard.

Harvesting Dandelion

Both the roots and the leaves of dandelion can be harvested. Regardless of which you are using, be sure to gather them from an area free of pesticides and lawn sprays. Be cautious even about harvesting from your own lawn unless you live away from traffic and are confident of the land's organic status.

Dandelion greens taste best when they're young and tender. As they grow, they become increasingly bitter. To harvest the roots, conversely, look for large plants. I've found it easiest to harvest the roots after a rainfall, when the ground is still soft and the roots come out whole.

Using Dandelion

Dandelion greens benefit both the urinary tract and liver, while the root works primarily on the liver. Most of the studies on the effectiveness of dandelion use dandelion root tinctures or dandelion root or leaf tea. In my experience, tinctures tend to be more potent than tea. Dandelion root is also available commercially in powdered or capsule form. You can make a decoction using two teaspoons of powdered dandelion root per cup of water. Bring to a boil and simmer for forty-five minutes. Make a large enough batch to ensure that it won't just evaporate during the cooking time. Drink one cup three times daily. Another option is to take one teaspoon of alcohol-based tincture three times daily.

Liver Regenerator

Dandelion root has been traditionally used in the treatment of liver disorders like jaundice, and increasing amounts of research support this use. Some health professionals recommend dandelion root tea for people taking antidepressant medications, since these drugs can impede the liver's detoxification pathways. Research in the *Journal of Medicinal Food* shows that dandelion also helps protect the liver against damage from other drugs, including painkillers like acetaminophen.[4]

If you plan to use the root to give your liver a boost, a typical dose is 500 to 2,000 mg of dandelion root in capsule form, taken daily for two weeks.

Blood Sugar Balancer and Diabetes Support

Dandelion contains a substance known as alpha-glucosidase, which is nature's blood-sugar reducer. It has been used for many years to treat diabetes. People with diabetes should work with a physician to monitor their blood sugar levels, because dandelion tea is so effective that it frequently helps people reduce their medications.

Energizer

In a study published in the journal *Molecules*, researchers found that animals given dandelion had a reduction in fatigue and a boost in immunity.[5]

Fat Burner

When it comes to weight loss, dandelion is virtually unmatched, in large part due to its effects on the liver. Dandelion root boosts liver function and increases the rate of fat metabolism in two ways: first, it stimulates the liver to produce more bile to send to the gallbladder, which helps burn fat, and second, it causes the gallbladder to contract and release its stored bile, further increasing fat metabolism. I usually recommend drinking it in tea form to aid weight loss. Not only can dandelion stimulate the liver to burn fat, it can also help reset our hormone balance so we stop storing as much fat, heal our cells to increase our energy levels, and speed up our metabolism so that weight melts off.

Anticancer Powerhouse

Dandelion's greatest therapeutic promise may lie in its ability to fight cancer. One of the most exciting studies about dandelion's anticancer properties was published in the journal *Evidence-Based Complementary and Alternative Medicine*. Canadian scientists found that after forty-eight hours of exposure to dandelion extract, cancer cells begin to die off. The study also found that dandelion was effective on cancer cells that were resistant to chemotherapy.[6] Another study, published in the *International Journal of Oncology*, found that a tea made from dandelion leaves decreased the growth of breast cancer cells, while a tea made from the root blocked the ability of cancer cells to invade healthy breast and prostate tissue.[7] In another study published in the online medical journal *PLoS One*, researchers found that an extract of dandelion root was able to selectively and efficiently kill cancer cells without toxicity to healthy cells. They concluded that natural products such as dandelion root have "great potential as non-toxic and effective alternatives to conventional modes of chemotherapy available today."[8] According to a study published in the journal *Molecular Carcinogenesis*, one of the ways that dandelion root seems to fight cancer is by making tumor cells more susceptible to the natural process known as apoptosis, which causes cells to essentially commit suicide. This study also found that dandelion root seems to increase the effectiveness of other cancer treatments used alongside it.[9]

Blood Purifier and Immune Booster

In a study published in *Advances in Hematology*, researchers found that dandelion significantly increased both red and white blood cell counts, making it a possible aid in the treatment of anemia, blood purification, and immune system modulation.[10]

Superbug Killer

Recently researchers have added the role of superbug killer to the dandelion's impressive health-boosting résumé, showing it to be effective against the bacteria *E. coli*, *Bacillus subtilis*, and MRSA.[11]

Osteoporosis Preventer

Next to cabbage, dandelion shoots (the stems, leaves, and flowers) have the highest amount of the bone-building mineral boron. According to James Duke, ten grams (just under seven tablespoons) of dried dandelion shoots provides over one milligram of boron and two hundred milligrams of calcium.[12] While that might sound like a lot of dandelion, keep in mind that drinking it as a tea makes it much easier to ingest. In addition, calcium in this form is much better absorbed than from other sources like dairy products.

Brain Food and Memory Enhancer

Dandelion flowers are one of the best sources of the nutrient lecithin, which, among other functions, increases the amount of the neurotransmitter acetylcholine and helps improve memory.[13]

Urinary Tract Infection Fighter

Dandelion root is a powerful diuretic, which means that it increases the production of urine. Increased urination helps flush out bladder bacteria, making dandelion root valuable in the treatment of bladder infections.

RECIPES

Roasted Dandelion Root "Coffee"

Chop raw dandelion root into small chunks, and roast it in a 200°F oven for 1 to 2 hours. Longer cooking times produce a darker roast taste. Remove from the oven, and allow the root to cool. Grind it in a high-powered blender or coffee grinder, and store in an airtight glass jar.

To use, add a tablespoon or two of the roasted root to almond or coconut milk with a dash of stevia (a naturally sweet herb that doesn't affect blood sugar levels), blend, and pour over ice. Or steep a tablespoon or two of roasted dandelion-root grounds in a cup of hot water.

Many health-food stores carry bulk dried dandelion root that you can roast and grind yourself, or you can buy roasted dandelion root to save time. Some health-food stores sell roasted and ground dandelion labeled as a coffee substitute.

Lemon-Garlic Dandelion Greens

Dandelion greens contain blood-building chlorophyll, which gives them their deep green color. They also contain bitter compounds that can help cleanse the liver. You can steam, sauté, or juice young dandelion greens. I love them chopped and sautéed with minced garlic and olive oil, then topped with fresh lemon juice and a dash of unrefined sea salt.

Super Health-Boosting Pumpkin-Spice Latte

This delicious pumpkin-spice latte is much lower in sugar than commercial varieties of the beverage and free of artificial ingredients. If you prefer a sweeter drink, simply increase the amount of coconut sugar used. You can serve it hot or iced, depending on your preference. Serves 2.

1 ½ cups almond or coconut milk
½ cup pumpkin purée
1 tablespoon roasted and ground dandelion root (see Roasted
    Dandelion Root "Coffee" recipe on page 60)
1 ½ tablespoons coconut sugar (or more to taste)
1 teaspoon ground cinnamon, plus more for sprinkling on top
⅛ teaspoon ground cloves
⅓ teaspoon ground nutmeg, plus more for sprinkling on top

Blend the almond or coconut milk, pumpkin purée, dandelion root, coconut sugar, cinnamon, cloves, and nutmeg together in a blender until smooth and creamy. To serve iced, pour over ice, sprinkle with additional cinnamon and nutmeg, and serve. To serve warm, heat in a small saucepan over medium to high heat until desired temperature has been reached. Sprinkle with additional cinnamon and nutmeg, and serve immediately.

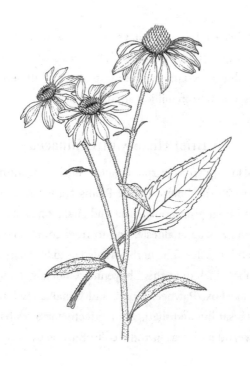

9. Echinacea

Echinacea purpurea, Echinacea angustifolia

W ho hasn't turned to this stunning beauty for help preventing or fighting off a nasty virus or to shorten the time spent suffering from a cold or flu? Echinacea has become the go-to herb for just such occasions for good reason: it works. Native Americans have known this for centuries. This herb's therapeutic reputation hasn't always been so glowing. Early in the last century, the *Journal of the American Medical Association* described the herb as a useless quack remedy. But when I started writing this herb profile, there were over two thousand scientific studies on echinacea. Few herbs have received so much scientific attention.[1] And consumers have endorsed echinacea's effectiveness: sales of echinacea products account for over 10 percent of all herb sales in the United States, about $100 million annually.

A Brief History of Echinacea

Echinacea, also known as purple coneflower, is a beautiful flowering plant native to North America. The Plains Native Americans used it medicinally to treat poisonous insect and snake bites, as an antiseptic to clean wounds, as an analgesic, and to treat communicable diseases like mumps and measles. The herb was also used by many other native American tribes, including the Cheyenne, Choctaw, Comanche, Dakota, Meskwaki Fox, Pawnee, Sioux, and Omaha.[2] Echinacea's combination of versatility and therapeutic effectiveness probably explains why this powerful herb was introduced to Europe by early travelers.

Growing Echinacea

Echinacea grows in conditions ranging from full sun to partial shade, as long as the soil is well drained and slightly alkaline. Echinacea seeds can be started indoors under warm lights in late winter or in a greenhouse in early spring. It can be sown directly outdoors in spring or late summer, toward the end of the growing season. Germination, which takes ten to twenty days, depends on light, so seeds should be covered with no more than a quarter inch of soil and kept moist. Echinacea is a perennial.

Seeds should be planted about twelve to eighteen inches apart, since the mature plants can reach four feet in height and often grow in clumps. Echinacea is a relatively low-maintenance plant but needs regular watering during dry conditions or in areas with low precipitation (less than an inch a week). It likes to be the star and thrives when weeds are removed and other plants are not crowding its space.

Echinacea reaches maturity in roughly 180 days, at which point you can harvest flowers, leaves, stems, and seeds. Don't forget to let the butterflies and bees enjoy the purple flowers for a while! When the flowers die back in the fall (after the first frost in cooler climates), the heads turn black and dry out. To harvest seeds, snip off the stem a few inches below the head, and shake the seeds into a container or paper bag. Don't worry if a few seeds fall on the ground: chances are they will self-sow and create more beautiful coneflowers next year.

Harvesting Echinacea

Echinacea roots should be left to mature for three to four years before they are harvested. You can dig up the plants in the fall, much as you would dig up potatoes from your vegetable patch, being careful not to pierce or damage the roots. Remove just a few roots from each plant, leaving enough behind to allow the plant to continue growing. Echinacea is increasingly considered an endangered plant, so growing it yourself gives this plant a needed boost.

Using Echinacea

Several species of Echinacea have medicinal benefits: two of the most effective and commonly used are *Echinacea angustifolia* and *Echinacea purpurea*.

Respiratory Relief

Research in the medical journal *Advances in Therapy* found that echinacea extracts significantly reduce the risk of recurring respiratory infections, ear infections, tonsillitis, and pharyngitis.[3] Echinacea has also been shown to reduce the severity of symptoms of respiratory infections. In one study published in the journal *Cell Immunology*, researchers found that echinacea demonstrated potent anti-inflammatory properties that are likely responsible for these effects.[4]

Lymph Lover

Most people have heard of echinacea as a cold or flu remedy or as an herbal immune system booster, but it is also a powerful lymphatic system cleanser. The lymphatic system is a network of nodes, tubules, fluid, and glands that "sweeps" toxins, wastes, and by-products of inflammation out of body tissues. In my twenty-five years of experience, I've found that a congested lymphatic system is almost always involved in pain. So if you're suffering from pain of any kind, it's a good idea to add a lymph-boosting herb like echinacea to your daily regimen. It is particularly effective combined with other lymph cleansers like astragalus, pokeroot, and wild indigo. (Note that pokeroot is best left to advanced herbalists.) Echinacea helps reduce congestion and swelling and get the lymph fluid moving. Make a decoction using two teaspoons of dried herb per cup of water. Bring to a boil. Simmer for fifteen minutes. Drink one cup three times per day. Alternatively, take one teaspoon of tincture three times per day.

Carpal Tunnel Syndrome Soother

New research in the *International Journal of Immunopathology and Pharmacology* found that echinacea combined with alpha lipoic acid, conjugated linoleic acid, and quercetin effectively reduced pain and other symptoms and also improved function in people suffering from carpal tunnel syndrome.[5]

Bug Bite Reliever

Summer brings hot weather, sun, flowers, picnics, and insects. Insects seem to love me, so I really wanted to find a natural remedy that takes the itch out of bug bites. After trying many remedies, I found echinacea to be the most effective. A tincture of echinacea applied directly to the bug bite quickly alleviates the itching and swelling, probably through its proven immune system balancing and anti-inflammatory properties.

Anti-inflammatory and Anti-pain Antidote

Echinacea has a long history of use for reducing inflammation. Its effectiveness was demonstrated not only in the *Cell Immunology* study cited above but also in another study published in the online medical journal *PLoS One*. In the latter study, researchers found that echinacea was able to regulate various types of chemicals that form in the body in response to pain and inflammation, suggesting it has potential for the treatment of disorders involving these symptoms.[6]

Insulin Resistance and Diabetes Treatment

Few people know about echinacea's potential uses for managing diabetes and the prediabetic syndrome known as insulin resistance. Research published in the journal *Planta Medica* found that echinacea showed significant antidiabetic effects because of its ability to regulate insulin metabolism and glucose.[7] Although research on Echinacea's antidiabetic effects is still in its infancy, this study suggests impressive potential.

RECIPE

Immune Booster Tea

Give your immune system a boost with this simple tea recipe. You can add a touch of honey or the natural sweetener stevia if you prefer a sweeter tea. If you're still not wild about the taste of this herbal tea, you can also add one teaspoon of dried peppermint while brewing.

> 1 teaspoon dried echinacea (flowers, leaves, stems, or seeds)
>   or 1 tablespoon fresh echinacea
> 1 cup water

In a small saucepan, boil the water. Stir in the echinacea flowers, and let the mixture steep for 10 to 15 minutes, uncovered. Strain. Drink one to three cups daily for best results.

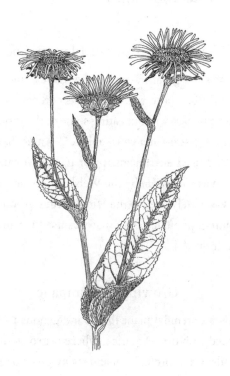

10. Elecampane

Inula helenium

Few people have ever heard of elecampane, yet as this herb proves itself powerful in healing more and more conditions, it is just a matter of time until elecampane takes its rightful place in the spotlight. It is a striking plant, growing to four or five feet tall and sporting large yellow flowers that look like a cross between dandelion heads and sunflowers. As its Latin name suggests, it is a rich source of the compound known as inulin. Inulin is a prebiotic found in some plants that nourishes beneficial microbes in the intestines.

A Brief History of Elecampane

Elecampane was in great favor in the Greek and Roman world: Dioscorides and Pliny both wrote about its potency as medicine. Pliny wrote: "Let no day pass without eating some of the roots of Enula, considered to help digestion and cause mirth."[1] Anglo-Saxons frequently wrote about and used elecampane prior to the Norman Conquest. It was also known as *marchalan* by the Welsh physicians of the thirteenth century and was widely used in the Middle Ages. About fifty years ago, it was made into a popular candy that was used for alleviating asthma and lung conditions.[2]

Growing Elecampane

Elecampane is a perennial plant that is indigenous to Europe but has been introduced to North America, where it grows freely in pastures and along roadsides. It prefers wet and rocky ground. The plant grows well in gardens provided that it has shade and is watered regularly. It prefers loamy or sandy, well-drained soil and moisture. It can be germinated from seed indoors or sown directly in gardens in the spring. It can also be propagated from the roots, provided the root pieces are at least two inches long and planted about a foot underground. Leave about ten inches between plants so they'll have room to grow. Keep the area free of weeds, and dig up some of the roots for use after at least two years of growth. This practice actually helps promote new plant growth.

Harvesting Elecampane

To use elecampane medicinally, dig up the roots in the fall and dry and grind them, or make them into a tincture following the instructions on page 16.

Using Elecampane

Breast Cancer Tumor Destroyer

In a recent study published in the medical journal *Phytotherapy Research*, scientists assessed the ability of hundreds of herbal extracts to prevent breast cancer tumors from growing. Elecampane root extract proved to be one of the most potent. It effectively stopped cancer cells from dividing, thereby inhibiting tumor growth.[3]

Native American Lung Healer

Elecampane has been used by Native Americans for many years to clear out excess mucus that impairs lung function. It is known as a natural antibacterial agent for the lungs, particularly effective for people who are prone to infections like bronchitis.[4] It can also help eliminate toxins from the lungs. Herbal practitioners often recommend one teaspoon of the herb per cup of boiling water, drunk three times daily for two to three weeks, or one dropperful of elecampane extract three times a day for the same period.

Probiotic Enhancer

The inulin contained in elecampane is one of the favorite foods of probiotics, including *Bifidobacteria* and *Lactobacillus*. Colonies of these beneficial bacteria in the gut help stave off infections, prevent inflammation, and encourage healthy bowels.

Liver Detoxifier

The liver has over five hundred functions, one of which is to cleanse the blood of toxic compounds found in food or the environment. Research published in the *Journal of Medicinal Food* found that compounds in elecampane boost the enzymes linked to this function.[5]

Tuberculosis Inhibitor

In 1885, an herbal authority known as Korab showed that elecampane was especially effective in killing tuberculosis bacteria. He showed that only a few drops of one of its compounds added to water could kill any bacteria present.[6] He was clearly on to something, since modern research published in the journal *Planta Medica* found that elecampane significantly inhibited the growth of *Mycobacterium tuberculosis* — the bacterium responsible for the serious and often deadly disease. This is good news considering that tuberculosis has made a recent comeback.[7] Elecampane is also helpful in treating other respiratory disorders, including asthma, emphysema, and whooping cough. It alleviates fever while battling infection and maximizing the excretion of toxins through perspiration. If you have a cough or bronchitis, elecampane may help.

Digestion Enhancer

In addition to promoting the health of the respiratory tract, elecampane also helps a sluggish digestive system. Use one teaspoon of herb per cup of water in an infusion or one half to one teaspoon of tincture three times a day.

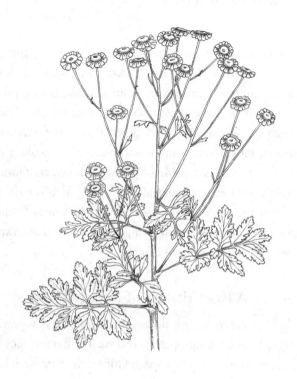

11. Feverfew

Tanacetum spp.

I have lived in two desert regions in Canada. Even many Canadians don't believe me when I tell them that there is desert in Canada, but the intense heat, the dry landscape, and the small cactus plants dotting the mountainsides (and sometimes my shoes) support my claim. The desert in Canada, however, supports a broader diversity of plants because it is only semiarid. During my first spring and summer in that area, I couldn't believe the number of feverfew plants popping up everywhere.

One of the things I've learned over my twenty-five years of

studying herbalism and natural medicine is that plants adapted to extreme conditions, such as drought, high altitude, heat, or cold, tend to have higher amounts of healing compounds. That's because the healing compounds are the same substances that ensure the plant's survival in these harsh conditions. When we ingest these compounds in food or as medicine, those same compounds impart their healing abilities to us. Feverfew, which is capable of growing in hot conditions with little water, is a most impressive healer. Not only does it have analgesic properties that can reduce the pain of migraines or arthritis, but it also reduces inflammation, stimulates digestion, and acts as an antispasmodic to help alleviate menstrual cramps.

A Brief History of Feverfew

Feverfew has been used as a medicine for millennia. It was particularly popular among Greek and European herbalists. The name comes from its history of use in treating fevers, though little modern research has been conducted on its use for this purpose. Nearly two thousand years ago, the Greek doctor Dioscorides recommended feverfew for "all hot inflammations."[1] The plant is believed to have originated in the Balkan Peninsula but is now found throughout Europe, Asia, Australia, North Africa, the United States, and Canada, primarily in fields or along roadsides. It is believed that the species name, *parthenium*, comes from its reputation for having saved the life of a worker who fell during the construction of the Parthenon in Greece in the fifth century BCE.[2] Additionally, the Kallawaya natives of the Andes mountains use feverfew for the treatment of kidney pain, colic, morning sickness, and stomachaches.

Growing Feverfew

Feverfew is fairly easy to grow from seed and can be grown indoors or outdoors in pots or in your garden. As you may have gathered, feverfew loves sunlight, and after it takes hold, it needs little care or attention. Its thick green foliage and small daisy-like flowers make it a great addition to any garden. To grow it from seed, simply sprinkle the seeds onto the soil and press down slightly to ensure that the seeds are in contact with the soil; there is no need to cover them. The best method is to start seeds in pots indoors and spray them with water rather than pouring water over them. This ensures the right amount of moisture for the seedlings to thrive. Grow them under a grow light or in a sunny windowsill for the first two weeks, and then plant the seedlings outdoors after the first frost. The plant grows to about a foot and a half to two feet tall and blooms all summer. If you cut the plant back in the fall, it will grow back in the spring.

Harvesting Feverfew

The aerial parts of the plant (those parts that are above the ground) are used in herbal medicine. To harvest feverfew, simply chop off the stems a couple of inches above the base, wash, and hang upside down to dry; or chop the leaves, flowers, and stems and prepare as a tea or tincture, following the instructions on pages 12 and 16.

Using Feverfew

Feverfew is a popular and proven remedy for migraine headaches, a particularly excruciating form of headache that is often characterized by knifing pain in one eye. But it is an all-around great pain reliever.

Using feverfew requires some caution. If you are allergic to ragweed, you may also be allergic to feverfew. Pregnant or nursing women should avoid feverfew. The prescription blood thinner warfarin (Coumadin) can interact with feverfew, so it is best not to take both together. Additionally, if you routinely take over-the-counter painkillers, it is best to skip feverfew. Also avoid taking it for a couple of weeks prior to undergoing surgery.

Headache and Migraine Reliever

Feverfew works best against migraines when taken regularly as a preventive measure. Some people assume that feverfew doesn't work when they take it after the onset of a migraine in an effort to quell the pain. But taking it similarly to migraine medications or over-the-counter pain relievers, after the onset of pain, is rarely effective. In a meta-analysis of studies using feverfew for the treatment of migraines published in the *Cochrane Database of Systematic Reviews*, researchers concluded that well-constructed studies of feverfew showed that it could reduce the prevalence of migraines.[3] Preventive use is also effective at reducing the incidence and severity of headaches in chronic headache sufferers.

Neuropathy Pain Reliever

Neuropathy is a general term used to describe disorders of the nervous system that cause pain, weakness, and numbness. It is a possible side effect of cancer chemotherapy. In a study published in the journal *Phytomedicine*, researchers found that feverfew was as effective as the drug gabapentin (an antiepileptic drug that has also been found to alleviate neuropathic pain).[4] Interestingly, the scientists who conducted the study found significant improvement in nerve-related pain when an extract of the flowers was used but none when the leaves were used, yet many feverfew products are made primarily from the leaves. The feverfew flower extract reduced neuropathy caused by the chemotherapy drug oxaliplatin and the antiviral drug dideoxycytidine.

Dermatitis Healer

Dermatitis is a medical term for any type of skin irritation that involves inflammation. Preliminary research has found that feverfew is helpful against dermatitis. It appears to work by healing damaged skin cells and reducing inflammation.[5]

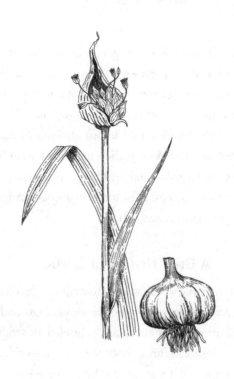

12. Garlic

Allium sativum

I remember a long-distance call with my mother a few years ago during which she continually bragged about my three-year-old nephew. She was telling me how much he still enjoyed being cuddled and then paused. "But," she said, "frequently the smell of garlic coming off of him is overwhelming. He just loves the stuff!" My nephew has eaten a raw-foods diet since he started on solid food, and he is one of the healthiest kids I know. Instinctively he knew that garlic was one of the world's superfoods.

Garlic lovers already know how good this member of the Liliaceae family tastes in myriad preparations. (If you are not a fan of garlic, chances are you just haven't tried it in a way that suits your taste buds.) But garlic can also help fend off flu viruses, lower blood pressure, prevent hardening of the arteries, and lessen cholesterol buildup in the heart. Thanks to many studies on garlic's medicinal properties, we also know that it has antibacterial and antifungal properties. Its pungent aroma, potent flavor, and powerful medicinal qualities make garlic a great choice for your garden and diet.

A Brief History of Garlic

Garlic may be the original wonder drug. Remains of the plant have been found in caves used by humans ten thousand years ago, and a Sumerian clay tablet dating from 3000 BCE contains a chiseled prescription for garlic.[1] Its use was widespread throughout the ancient world, from southern Europe to China, and it was revered by both the Egyptians and the Greeks for its ability to ward off disease and increase strength.[2] Over the past century, scientists have confirmed the medicinal properties of garlic through numerous studies that have illustrated its effectiveness against diverse fungal, bacterial, viral, and yeast strains. During World War I, garlic was used to treat wounded soldiers' infections as well as amoebic dysentery.[3]

Growing Garlic

Affectionately known as "the stinking rose" for obvious reasons, garlic comprises a multisegmented bulb, each segment of which is called a clove, and thin green leaves that typically grow between one and two feet tall. At the height of summer, small white or pink flowers appear. A study conducted by the U.S. Department of Agriculture's National Center for Genetic Resources Preservation assessed 211 varieties of garlic, including *Allium longicuspis*, a wild garlic found in Central Asia from which *Allium sativum* is descended. The study confirmed that there is substantial diversity in chemical composition within the garlic family.[4]

For the home gardener and consumer, the main difference is between "hard-neck" and "soft-neck" types of garlic.[5] The former are considered more aromatic and flavorful; they grow scapes, edible flower stalks. Soft-neck types are commonly sold in grocery stores because of their longer shelf life. Both are easy to grow and are a wonderful addition to any garden.

Like the onion, scallion, leek, chive, and shallot, to which it is related, garlic likes full sun but not intense heat, high humidity, or heavy rainfall. New garlic plants need regular moisture to develop their roots; however, once they are established, the plants thrive in rich, loose, well-drained soil.[6] Hard-neck varieties tend to fare better in colder climates.[7]

Garlic can be planted in early spring or mid-autumn, prior to the first frost. Push bulbs into the soil approximately two inches deep and six inches apart. If you are growing rows of garlic, leave about a foot between rows.[8] Do not overwater garlic, or you risk rotting the bulbs.

Harvesting Garlic

Harvesting times vary based on the season of planting and the climate of your area. As the leaves begin to turn brown, check a few plants to see if they are mature. The change of color usually means the garlic is ready. Keep the leaves on the plant, wash the dirt off the bulbs, and let them dry in a warm, sunny place. Once they are thoroughly dry, you can string them together and store them in a well-ventilated area with low humidity.[9]

Using Garlic

Like most plant-based foods, garlic offers more nutritional and medicinal properties in its raw state. Studies have shown that the beneficial compounds in garlic can be destroyed or broken down faster when it is cooked or processed.[10] Thus recipes that use uncooked or lightly cooked garlic provide more benefit. Salad dressings, for example, are a great way to fit raw garlic into your diet.

Superfood and Super Flavor Enhancer

There are very few savory dishes that don't benefit from the addition of garlic. Cooking or roasting garlic helps mellow both its flavor and its aroma to enhance soups, stews, stir-fries, curries, sauces, and pastas. It is a staple in many European and Asian cuisines and is growing in popularity in North America. The proliferation of garlic-themed restaurants and food shops is a testament to its diverse and delicious contribution to our diet.

Most of the garlic on our grocery-store shelves comes from California and is likely of the Creole variety. Italian or Mexican garlic is a bit smaller than the Creole and has a slightly purplish-colored skin. Tahitian garlic is also known as elephant garlic because of its large size. But when it comes to garlic, good things come in small packages: the Italian or Mexican variety is the most potent.

When buying garlic, look for garlic that is firm and free of black mildew on the skin. Store it at room temperature in a well-ventilated spot such as a garlic keeper. Most experts suggest eating at least one clove a day to reap the maximum health benefits. If your taste buds shout for more, let them have it.

Germ Buster Extraordinaire

According to James Duke, botanist and author of *The Green Pharmacy*, the common cold is caused by any of more than two hundred viruses.[11] He points out that garlic contains several compounds that can battle colds and flu, including allicin, a powerful natural broad-spectrum antibiotic.[12]

Cancer Fighter

Allicin is not only a natural antibiotic; it is also an antioxidant that helps to prevent the cell damage that can be a precursor of cancer.[13]

Researchers have concluded that garlic has the ability to inhibit differ-ent types of tumors and lower the risks of esophageal, stomach, and prostate cancers.[14] Research has also shown that allicin can not only slow the proliferation of human gastric cancer cells but also cause can-cer cell death.[15]

RECIPES

Savory Lentil Bowl

Don't underestimate how good these simple ingredients can be when combined. This recipe is a snap to make and a great way to add more garlic and beans to your diet. And it's also a great way to boost your fiber intake!

Serves 2 to 4.

2 tablespoons extra-virgin olive oil
2 medium or 3 small onions, chopped
3 cups cooked lentils, drained
1 garlic clove, minced
1 teaspoon unrefined sea salt

Heat the oil over medium-low heat in a large skillet, making sure it never smokes. Add the onions and sauté them over medium-low heat until lightly browned, about 10 to 15 minutes. Place in a medium bowl, and add the lentils, garlic, and salt; mix well. Serve warm.

Ginger Chili Quinoa

I was tired of quinoa recipes that all tasted alike, so I developed this spicy Asian-inspired recipe, and now it's my favorite way to eat this superfood. It's packed with flavor and anti-inflammatory ginger and cayenne, making it the perfect detox dinner.

Serves 2 to 4.

1 cup quinoa, rinsed
1¾ cups water
1 small garlic clove, minced
1 small fresh cayenne chili, minced
½ teaspoon unrefined sea salt
One 1-inch piece fresh ginger, peeled and minced
1 small onion, chopped
1 tablespoon coconut oil

Mix all ingredients in a small saucepan. Cover, place on medium-high heat, and bring to a boil. Stir, cover, and reduce the heat to its lowest setting; allow the quinoa to simmer for 20 minutes or until all the water is absorbed. Fluff with a fork and serve.

Savory Garlic Salad Dressing

This is one of my favorite salad dressings. It's delicious served over salad greens like romaine lettuce or tossed with cooked greens like kale or collard. Either way, it makes greens taste amazing. Enjoy.

Makes approximately 1 cup.

½ cup extra-virgin olive oil
Juice of one lemon (approximately 3 tablespoons)
1 clove garlic, minced
1 teaspoon Dijon mustard
⅓ cup white wine vinegar
1 teaspoon unrefined sea salt
Dash of freshly cracked pepper
Dash of cayenne pepper

Blend all ingredients together until smooth and creamy.

Garlicky Greens

One of the most common questions I am asked is, "How can I cook greens to make them taste good?" Every time I give people this recipe, they come back and tell me they can't believe how good it is. Somehow the combination of garlic and lemon juice makes greens taste fantastic. You can make this dish with spinach, kale, collard greens, beet greens, or any other type of leafy greens. Kale is a good choice because it is packed with calcium and other minerals and grows easily even in northern climates. It also contains a fair amount of fiber and is packed with chlorophyll too.

Makes approximately 3 cups.

1 tablespoon coconut oil or extra-virgin olive oil
1 large bunch kale (or another type of leafy greens, if you prefer), washed and coarsely chopped
1 clove garlic, minced
Juice of 1 lemon
Dash of unrefined salt

In a large frying pan with a lid, heat the oil, being careful not to allow it to smoke. Add the greens to the pan with a small amount of water. Cover. Once the greens have turned a bright shade of green and have softened, add the garlic and sauté for an additional minute or two. Remove from the heat, and toss the greens with the fresh lemon juice and salt. Serve immediately.

Roasted Garlic

For those of you scared to offend the significant other in your life, try roasting whole garlic to tame its pungency. Cut off the stem, exposing the top of each clove, and drizzle a bit of olive oil over it. Wrap it in foil or place it in a garlic roaster, and bake at 350°F for about an hour. This greatly minimizes the powerful garlic aroma but creates a spread that tastes fabulous and has the consistency of butter. Spread on bread, add to soups or stews, or blend with a little olive oil and wine vinegar for a delicious salad dressing.

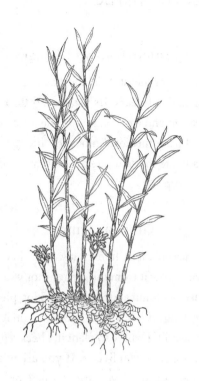

13. Ginger

Zingiber officinale

For most people, the mention of ginger calls to mind gingersnaps or gingerbread. But ginger is more than just a holiday baking favorite, particularly when it comes to the fresh root. It is among my favorite natural medicines, partly because I love the taste and the warmth it provides on cool days and partly because it is one of the best natural medicines available. Not only has it been found to be superior to pharmaceutical drugs for treating many conditions, but it has none of the horrible side effects and offers many health advantages to those who use it on a regular basis.

A Brief History of Ginger

Ginger originated in Southeast Asia and has been used in Ayurvedic medicine for thousands of years. Its use spread throughout the world with human migration and exploration. It was first used to make delicacies and sweets during medieval times. By the fourteenth century it had become so valuable that a moderate amount of ginger was worth the same as a live sheep.[1]

Growing Ginger

Growing this tropical plant at home may seem like an impossibility, but it's not. You can grow it from the ginger root you find at your local grocery store. Select a plump and healthy-looking piece of ginger root at least four inches long. If it has some green tips on it already, so much the better. Before deciding where to plant it, check a gardening manual to see which growing zone you live in. If you are in zone 7 or higher, you can grow ginger outside; if you are in zone 6 or lower, you'll need to grow it in a pot indoors, which is perfectly fine. Either way, it takes about ten months for ginger to mature. If you're growing it outdoors, add compost or manure to the soil. Plant the root no deeper than one inch in the ground in the early spring, after all signs of frost have passed. If you're growing it indoors, use a good potting soil. Don't worry if the root pushes back out of the ground as it grows. Water the ginger root thoroughly until there is evidence of a plant forming; then water deeply but infrequently.

Harvesting Ginger

Ginger root is ready to harvest the following spring after planting. Alternatively, you can wait until summer for a larger harvest. You can also save root sections that have any greenery attached and replant them for another year's harvest. Simply dig up the root and use it as you would any purchased fresh ginger root. It has so many culinary and medicinal uses that you'll always want to have a fresh supply on hand.

Using Ginger

Avoid using dried ginger, as the medicinal value is greatly diminished. Fresh is always best.

Nausea Remedy

While you may already be aware of ginger's use to alleviate nausea or motion sickness, you might not realize just how powerful it is for this purpose. Researchers published a study in the *Clinical Journal of Oncology Nursing* about ginger's ability to reduce the severe nausea and vomiting that often accompany cancer chemotherapy. They found that those people taking ginger had much less nausea and fewer vomiting episodes than those in the control group.[2]

Arthritis Reliever

A study published in the journal *Arthritis* compared ginger extract to the common drugs betamethasone (cortisone) and ibuprofen for the treatment of osteoarthritis and rheumatoid arthritis. One of the parameters measured in the study was the production of cytokines — immune-regulating substances that can have inflammatory effects on the body and that are therefore linked to pain. While ibuprofen is a popular arthritis pain remedy (under brand names such as Advil and Motrin), in this study it showed no effect on cytokine production. Both betamethasone and ginger extract reduced cytokines to comparable degrees. The authors of the study note that "ginger extract was as effective an anti-inflammatory agent as betamethasone."[3] While betamethasone has been used for decades to relieve pain and inflammation, it is also linked with many serious side effects, including vision problems, weight gain, swelling, shortness of breath, depression, seizures, pancreatitis, heart arrhythmias, muscle weakness, high blood pressure, severe headaches, anxiety, chest pains, sleep problems, acne, slow wound healing, and more. Ginger, however, is a powerful anti-inflammatory that is safe for use and confers many other health benefits as well.

Superior Joint-Pain Medication

Research by Krishna C. Srivastava, a world-renowned researcher on the therapeutic effects of spices at Odense University in Denmark, found that ginger is an effective pain remedy.[4] In one study, Dr. Srivastava gave people suffering from joint pain small amounts of ginger daily for three months. The majority of people experienced significant reductions in pain, swelling, and morning stiffness. Dr. Srivastava also found that ginger was superior to nonsteroidal anti-inflammatory drugs (NSAIDs) like Tylenol or Advil because NSAIDs only work at one level, by blocking the formation of inflammatory compounds. Ginger, on the other hand, not only blocks the formation of the inflammatory compounds — prostaglandins and leukotrienes — but also has antioxidant effects that reduce inflammation and acidity in the fluid within the joints.

Muscle Pain Remedy

The compounds found in ginger known as gingerols are well-established anti-pain compounds. Research published in the *Journal of Pain* further demonstrates that ginger is an effective natural anti-inflammatory that helps to reduce muscle pain.[5] In addition, ginger increases blood flow to the injured and inflamed area, thereby improving healing. Study participants ingested between five hundred and one thousand milligrams daily. The higher doses brought faster and more extensive relief. All participants who took ginger experienced some improvement, and none experienced any negative side effects, even those who took the high doses of ginger for over two years. Both raw ginger and heated ginger were used in the study with similar effectiveness.

Some studies suggest that eating ginger or taking a ginger supplement prior to strenuous exercise may reduce the resulting muscle pain.[6] Grated, fresh ginger can also be applied directly to the skin in a painful area. This stimulates circulation and reduces muscular pains and stiffness. However, it can irritate sensitive skin.

Potent Antiviral and Antibacterial Agent

More and more exciting research showcases ginger's potency against viruses and bacteria alike, even when antibiotic or antiviral drugs fail.[7] That's important news as we collectively cope with superbugs resistant to conventional drugs.

Possible Brain Health Protector

According to a study conducted by Honlei Chen and his colleagues at the Harvard School of Public Health, inflammation is implicated in the development of Parkinson's disease.[8] Interestingly, inflammatory processes are also known to play a role in the development of Alzheimer's disease. Therefore, foods that have an anti-inflammatory effect may help maintain a healthy brain and prevent brain disease. Additionally, ginger seems to prevent the reduction of a neurotransmitter known as dopamine involved in Parkinson's disease, suggesting two potential methods by which ginger may be helpful in the prevention or treatment of Parkinson's.[9]

Cholesterol and Stroke-Risk Reducer

Research shows that ginger reduces the level of harmful cholesterol in the blood, thereby reducing the risk of stroke. Researchers studied ninety-five people with high blood levels of triglycerides and LDL cholesterol (the "bad" cholesterol), and low levels of HDL ("good") cholesterol. They divided the participants into two groups: the first group took one thousand milligrams of ginger three times a day; the other group took a placebo. After forty-five days, participants taking the ginger showed a greater drop in LDL cholesterol and a greater increase in HDL cholesterol.[10]

Anticancer Protector

Ginger contains several compounds that have demonstrated anticancer and tumor-destroying properties, including gingerol, shogaol, paradol, and zerumbone. Research shows that ginger and its active ingredients help control colorectal, gastric, ovarian, liver, skin, breast, and prostate cancers.[11]

Blood Sugar Balancer and Diabetes Aid

A study showed that ginger significantly lowered blood sugar levels and LDL cholesterol, and raised HDL cholesterol in animals with diabetes, suggesting that the herb may offer potential as a natural diabetes treatment in humans.[12]

Gastrointestinal Soother

Ginger has shown great promise in an animal study for the treatment of gastrointestinal disorders like irritable bowel disease (IBD), Crohn's disease, colitis, and ulcers. High doses used in one study showed ginger to be as effective as the common drug sulfasalazine used to treat colitis, without the many harmful side effects.[13]

HOW TO REAP THE ANTI-PAIN BENEFITS OF GINGER

- Add chopped, fresh ginger to soups, stews, stir-fries, vegetable or meat dishes, and desserts. Ginger is delicious in many savory and sweet dishes.
- Add fresh ginger to a juicer while making juices. It combines well with many vegetables and fruits, such as carrots or apples.
- Ginger (*Zingiber officinale*) is available in capsules as a dietary supplement. Follow package directions.
- Chopped, fresh ginger can be added to water and boiled in a pot for forty-five minutes to an hour, then drunk as a hot or iced tea. Add a few drops of stevia (a naturally sweet, sugar-free herb) to sweeten.
- Take thirty drops of ginger tincture three times daily. (Avoid the alcohol extract if you are an alcoholic, suffering from liver disease, or diabetic.)

Medicine never tasted so good.

RECIPES

Asian Ginger Vinaigrette

I eat a lot of salads, so variety is important to me. This dressing helps keep salads interesting. I love the pungent flavor of ginger contrasted with the sweetness of the honey and rice vinegar and the sweet and savory taste of miso. Miso is a fermented paste made from soy (or sometimes brown rice) packed with enzymes that promote healing and digestion. This dressing can be made ahead and stored in a glass jar in the refrigerator for up to two weeks. Toss it with greens, grated vegetables of your choice, kelp noodles, or cooked spaghetti squash.

Makes about 1¼ cups.

⅔ cup extra-virgin olive oil (preferably a fruity-tasting one)
⅓ cup rice vinegar
2 heaping teaspoons miso
1 teaspoon raw, unrefined honey
1 tablespoon freshly grated ginger

Add all ingredients to a jar, cover, and shake. Or blend together using a blender, immersion blender, or handheld mixer.

Thai Ginger-Coconut Soup

This is one of my favorite soups. It is perfect for a cool autumn or winter dinner, but it's so good, and so easy, that you'll probably want to make it year-round. It takes about 45 minutes to prepare and cook, but the actual prep time is closer to 5 or 10 minutes.

Serves 2 to 4 as a main dish.

1 tablespoon coconut oil
1 cup brown rice
2 large carrots, chopped

2 stalks celery, chopped
1 large onion, chopped
3 cups water
Half of one fresh chili, minced, or ¼ teaspoon chili powder
One 2-inch piece of fresh ginger, chopped into matchsticks
1 organic chicken breast, sliced into bite-sized pieces
1 can coconut milk (choose the full-fat version, not low-fat)
Celtic sea salt or Himalayan crystal salt to taste

In a large pot or Dutch oven, melt the coconut oil over medium heat. Stir in the rice, carrots, celery, onion, water, chili, and ginger, and cover. Let the soup simmer gently over medium heat for 30 minutes. Add the chicken and coconut milk, and simmer for another 15 minutes. Add the salt. Serve immediately.

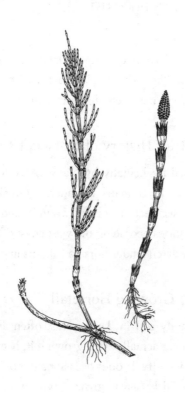

14. Horsetail

Equisetum arvense

Imagine going back in time to 400 million years ago, over 100 million years before dinosaurs roamed the earth. You might find yourself amid a stand of 300-foot-tall trees growing out of primordial swamp. Resting in these gigantic trees, you'd see enormous dragonflies with a two-foot wingspan eating fresh shoots from the trees.[1] The trees would be ancestors of the plant we know today as horsetail. It's hard to imagine that plants could withstand the Ice Age, but horsetail did, which is a testament to its strength and resilience.

What does this herb have to do with actual horses? Its Latin genus name, *Equisetum*, means "horse bristle," probably with reference to the long, thin leaves, whose shape resembles horsehair.

A Brief History of Horsetail

Horsetail has been used medicinally by Native Americans, Tibetans, and Chinese, as well as the Romans and ancient Greeks. It has been used to treat tuberculosis, heal ulcers and wounds, and halt bleeding. The Hesquiat First Nations people on the west coast of Vancouver Island have traditionally eaten tender horsetail shoots in early spring.[2]

Growing Horsetail

Horsetail grows in sandy soil in damp areas, often along riverbeds and lakeshores. I've never actually tried growing it, because it is fairly abundant and easy to identify. It does occasionally pop up in gardens, so I believe it would be fairly easy to grow. A type of plant that has survived 400 million years of life on Earth probably isn't that fussy. Like humans, neighboring plants obtain valuable nutrients from horsetail, especially silica.

Like ferns, horsetail reproduces via spores, and its roots can spread up to three feet underground. It prefers wet or boggy areas and sandy or poor soil. The plants prefer at least a half day of full sun and hot temperatures. But I've seen horsetail growing in places that are not particularly warm. It is best started from seed at least six weeks prior to the first frost and then transplanted outdoors. Water regularly.

Harvesting Horsetail

Horsetail can easily be dried by hanging it upside down or by laying it out in a thin layer on baking sheets and allowing it to air-dry for a couple of days. Fresh horsetail can be cut to make infusions or tinctures. Horsetail tincture was one of the first herbal medicines I made when I was getting started as an amateur forager and herbalist. Not only was it easy to identify in the forest, but the fact that it was fairly easy to distinguish from poisonous plants helped boost my confidence.

Using Horsetail

Time and again research has shown that plants adapted to survive in difficult conditions frequently contain phytochemicals that have medicinal value to humans. Horsetail's high silica content gives it an important role in the strengthening of arteries, skin, bones, cartilage, and connective tissues.

Bone, Nail, and Hair Builder

Silica is essential to building bone, strengthening the immune system, regulating calcium in the body, and building strong nails, hair, and teeth. A silica deficiency is linked with skin wrinkling, insomnia, irritability, muscle cramps, poor bone development, soft or brittle nails, and thinning or loss of hair. Replenishing your silica levels by using horsetail may bring an improvement in any of these symptoms, although it can take up to two months of regular use to see results. For a tea that improves the health of bones, nails, and hair, use one teaspoon of dried herb per cup of boiled water. Pour the water over the herb and let steep for about ten minutes. Strain. Drink three cups daily.

Osteoporosis Preventer

Researchers studied the effectiveness of horsetail in building bone and preventing infections that can be linked to fractures and osteoporosis. Published in the journal *Cell Proliferation*, the study showed that horsetail improved the bone-building ability of osteoblasts — cells that make bone by laying down a matrix to which minerals bind to form bone — while reducing the likelihood of infection. The scientists concluded that using horsetail extract may be a good bone-regeneration strategy.[3] Another study published in the same journal a few months later showed that horsetail inhibited the action of cells that break down bone, a process that contributes to conditions like osteoporosis.[4]

Anticancer Aid

Multiple studies suggest that horsetail may be helpful in treating cancer. In a study published in the *Journal of Medicinal Food*, scientists found that horsetail not only exhibited strong antioxidant properties but also showed the ability to halt the proliferation of cancer cells.[5] A study published in the *Bulletin of Experimental Biology and Medicine* found that a combination of horsetail, greater celandine, elecampane, and the mushroom chaga had the most potent antitumor effect of those substances tested on breast cancer.[6] Another study found that the same blend of herbs and mushroom had reduced the growth of lymphoma and leukemia tumors and increased survival rates by 33 percent in animals tested.[7] While the research on the use of horsetail to treat cancer is still in its infancy, the herb shows promise.

Wound Healer

Scientists assessed horsetail's reputation as a traditional wound healer by applying an ointment made with horsetail extract to diabetic wounds in animals. They found that the horsetail ointment exhibited significant wound-healing ability.[8]

RECIPE

Horsetail Skin-Healing Lotion

Horsetail is rich in silica, a key mineral for skin health that also helps heal damaged skin. This is a good all-purpose lotion that doesn't require a lot of ingredients and can be used for a wide variety of skin conditions on a daily basis.

Makes about 2 cups.

1 cup water

2 teaspoons dried horsetail (or 4 teaspoons fresh horsetail)

¾ cup sweet almond or apricot kernel oil

2 tablespoons shaved beeswax

Boil the water and pour it over the horsetail. Cover the mixture and let it brew for 10 to 20 minutes. Strain out the herb, reserving the horsetail-infused water. Set aside.

Pour the oil into a Pyrex measuring cup, and add the shaved beeswax. Set the measuring cup in a saucepan of water that reaches about halfway up the side of the measuring cup. Heat the mixture until the beeswax dissolves, and then remove the measuring cup from the heat immediately. Allow it to cool for a minute or two, but not longer, as the beeswax will begin to harden.

Pour the horsetail-infused water into a blender, cover, and begin blending it on high speed. With the blender running, slowly pour the beeswax mixture through the hole in the blender lid. The mixture will begin to thicken after about three-quarters of the beeswax has been incorporated.

Once all the beeswax has been blended, immediately pour the lotion into one 16-ounce glass jar or two 8-ounce glass jars. Use a spatula to remove any remaining lotion from the blender.

The lotion lasts about 3 months and is best kept in the fridge, since it contains no artificial preservatives.

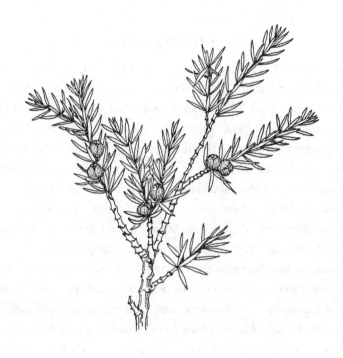

15. Juniper

Juniperus communis

On a cool, crisp autumn afternoon hiking in the magnificent Canadian Rocky Mountains, my husband, Curtis, remarked on the scent of juniper wafting through the pure mountain air. Thousands of juniper plants with indigo-blue berries blanketed the earth around our feet. With every step we took, the rich, clean aroma of juniper intensified. We stopped to collect a small basketful of the beautiful little juniper berries to enjoy later as a refreshing tea or an ingredient in sauerkraut. Years later, the delightful scent of juniper still transports me back to that blissful day in the Rockies.

A Brief History of Juniper

Juniper berries have been found in ancient Egyptian tombs, including the tomb of the pharaoh Tutankhamen, suggesting that the berries had spiritual importance. The ancient Greeks used juniper berries as medicine and medicinal food. Their athletes used them in preparation for Olympic events, believing that the berries increased physical stamina.[1] Juniper also has a long history of use as a food and drink ingredient in Europe, where it grows abundantly. Juniper berries give gin its unique and distinct flavor, and are used in fermented foods like sauerkraut, both as a seasoning and as a probiotic booster for fermentation, because of the white "bloom" that appears on uncooked juniper berries. In North America, juniper berries were widely used by the Cree as a diuretic. The leaves were dried and dusted over sores, and the root was made into an infusion to treat kidney stones. Other native peoples, including the Kwakiutl, boiled juniper for a full day until it produced a gum-like substance, which was used in decoctions to treat shortness of breath and to purify the blood. Some Native American tribes have also used the seeds inside juniper berries as beads for jewelry and decoration.[2] Juniper has also been used in the practice of voodoo in Louisiana.[3]

Growing Juniper

There are 170 different species of juniper. The most common is *Juniperus communis* (hence the name); other common species include *J. drupacea*, *J. phoenicea*, *J. oxycedrus*, *J. deppeana*, *J. occidentalis*, and *J. californica*. One variety, *Juniperus sabina*, is toxic and should not be consumed. Juniper is hardy and easy to grow except in extreme cold and heat. Even so, it seems to thrive in the extreme winter cold of the Canadian Rockies. The growth habits of the various species range from low-lying shrubs to tall trees. In your garden, any species is likely to thrive unless it is overwatered or in deep shade. Juniper prefers full sunlight and well-drained, slightly acidic soil, although it will grow in most soil, including saline coastal soils. When planting juniper, as for any shrub or tree, dig a hole twice the size of the root ball, add some compost, and plant the juniper, tamping down the soil. Water two to three times weekly for the first few weeks. After that, juniper rarely needs watering except in severe drought conditions.

Harvesting Juniper

Juniper, like apples, blueberries, cabbage, grapes, and plums, has a white substance on the outer leaves or skin. This is a natural bloom of beneficial microorganisms that help encourage the fermentation process when making sauerkraut or naturally fermented pickles. When harvesting any of these fruits and vegetables for use in fermented foods, don't wash or wipe off all of this bloom.

Using Juniper

Juniper berries are mildly cleansing and restorative of the kidneys. Juniper is also effective for arthritis and rheumatism as well as generalized muscular and joint pain. Use one teaspoon of dried juniper berries per cup of boiling water. Allow to infuse for at least ten minutes. Drink one cup three times daily. Alternatively, take one teaspoon of tincture three times daily, or take as directed on the package.

Be sure to work with an herbalist if you use juniper, because the berries can be toxic in large amounts. Avoid taking juniper if you have kidney disease or while pregnant or lactating. Do not use for prolonged periods. Avoid making an extract of the *Juniperus sabina*, as this species of juniper is toxic when ingested.

Urinary Tract Infection Fighter

Juniper's antimicrobial action (it has shown activity against bacteria, fungi, and viruses in studies) and its diuretic properties make juniper a potent remedy for urinary tract infections. An infusion, a tincture, or a seasoning made of ground dried juniper berries is best for this purpose.

Alzheimer's Aid

While most therapeutic applications of juniper use the berries, preliminary research has assessed the effects of an extract made from the leaves and shoots. They showed significant antioxidant activity and the ability to inhibit an enzyme known as cholinesterase, which is involved in the progression of Alzheimer's disease, suggesting that juniper may have a role to play in preventing or treating the disease.[4]

Possible Parkinson's Treatment

Another study in the journal *Neurochemical Research* found that inhalation of the volatile oils of the juniper plant significantly reduced the activity of acetylcholinesterase (the primary form of cholinesterase). This effect could account for the results mentioned above, but it also means that juniper may hold promise for the treatment of Parkinson's disease, dementia, and glaucoma.[5]

RECIPES

Urinary Tract Healing Tea

This tea is good for fighting urinary tract infections or for giving the urinary tract an occasional boost if you're prone to infections. To make an infusion, lightly crush one teaspoon of fresh or dried juniper berries, pour one cup of boiling water over them, cover, and allow the mixture to sit for 20 minutes. Strain the liquid, then drink. Use three times daily.

Apple Juniper Sauerkraut

This delicious sauerkraut is a favorite in my home. My husband, Curtis, enjoys it so much that I jokingly started calling him Krautis. Not only is sauerkraut delicious, but it is easy to make, and it's packed with health-building probiotics that are usually lacking in store-bought kraut. The recipe is long simply because I've included detailed directions for those new to making fermented foods.

Making probiotic-rich vegetable dishes usually involves soaking the vegetables in a saltwater solution (brining). The brine draws water out of the vegetables and kills the microorganisms that decompose food while allowing probiotics, like *Lactobacillus*, to survive. At one time pickles were made in brine and were rich in probiotics. Today, the pickles sold in grocery stores are usually made with white vinegar, are loaded with sugar, have not undergone any fermentation process, and usually contain chemical preservatives. Thus they lack probiotics. Making your own pickles yields a much healthier product.

You can use a variety of fermentation vessels, including stoneware crocks, ceramic or glass bowls, and wide-mouthed mason jars. Avoid using metal or plastic containers, as the acid produced by the fermentation process can react chemically with these materials. In addition, most beneficial microbes do not grow well in a metal container.

Whatever container you use, you'll need a plate, jar, or cover that fits inside it. This is used to keep the vegetables submerged in the brine; if they float up and are exposed to air, they may spoil. I use a plate as large as I can find. Flea markets and antique shops are great places to find both crocks and plates of different sizes. You'll also need to place a weight on top of the plate to keep it in position. A one-gallon glass jug works well as a weight for larger crocks, and mason jars filled with water make good weights for smaller crocks or bowls.

As it ferments, this delicious sauerkraut turns a brilliant pink color that is a gorgeous addition to any plate. Enjoy it on its own as a delicious condiment; on salad, hot dogs, sausages, or burgers; or over a bowl of brown or black rice. Add it to sandwiches and wraps, or serve as a side dish.

Makes approximately 2 quarts.

2 small to medium heads of green cabbage, shredded
2 teaspoons juniper berries, coarsely cracked in a mortar and
    pestle (or using a hammer, with the juniper berries placed
    between two clean tea towels)
3 medium apples, sliced

3 tablespoons unrefined fine sea salt, or 6 tablespoons unrefined
coarse sea salt (do not use iodized salt, as it can interfere with
the fermentation process)

1 quart filtered water (preferably unchlorinated water, as the
chlorine can interfere with the fermentation process)

Place a thick layer of the cabbage at the bottom of a large, clean
crock or bowl, pushing down with your fist or a wooden spoon to release the juices. Add a sprinkling of juniper berries, followed by a layer
of apples. Push down on the mixture again to release more juices. Continue layering, and pressing to remove juices, until all the cabbage, juniper, and apples have been added.

In a pitcher or large measuring cup, dissolve the sea salt in the
water, stirring to encourage the salt to dissolve. Pour the liquid over the
cabbage mixture until the ingredients are submerged, leaving a couple
of inches of room at the top for the ingredients to expand.

Place a plate inside the crock on top of the cabbage mixture, and
then weigh it down with food-safe weights or a bowl or jar of water.
Cover with a lid or cloth. Leave the mixture to ferment for at least a
week, checking periodically to ensure that the vegetables are still completely submerged.

If any mold forms on the surface of the liquid, simply scoop it out.
It will not spoil the sauerkraut. It may form where the mixture meets
the air but not deeper inside the crock.

After one week, or longer if preferred, dish out the sauerkraut into
jars or a bowl, and store in the refrigerator, where it will last for at least
a few months. I allow my sauerkraut to ferment for at least two weeks
to develop the classic sauerkraut taste.

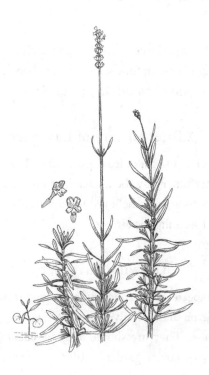

16. Lavender

Lavandula angustifolia

I visited an organic lavender farm last summer. From half a mile down the road, I could smell the aroma wafting through the air. The rolling hillside was covered with the stunning silvery-green and purple lavender plants. I felt immediately transported to a peaceful, relaxed state. How much of this feeling was linked to the aromatic effects of lavender and how much to the natural beauty of this lovely environment, I'll never know. Either way, it was an experience to remember.

You can easily experience the beauty and healing properties of lavender by growing your own for use in food and body care. It will grow happily indoors in pots or outside in your garden.

A Brief History of Lavender

Lavender has been in use for at least 2,500 years. It was used for mummification and perfumery by the ancient Egyptians, Phoenicians, and Arabs. The Romans are also believed to have used lavender for cooking, bathing, and scenting the air.

Growing Lavender

There are many species of lavender, most ranging from one to two feet tall and forming mounds of silver-green foliage topped with purple flowers in summer. They are simple to grow, making them an ideal plant for the lazy or novice gardener. I live in a semiarid climate, and even if I forget to water lavender for weeks, it still grows. Shorter varieties make a stunning edging along walkways, while taller kinds make beautiful, scented hedges.

Lavender grows best in a sunny location with well-drained soil. Pay attention to the spacing recommendations when purchasing lavender plants, as some varieties can grow to a few feet in diameter. You can also grow lavender from seed. It needs regular watering to get started but only infrequent watering after the plant takes hold.

Harvesting Lavender

To harvest, wait until the plant blooms, and cut the stems about one-third of the way from the flower heads. Place the cut lavender in a vase or pitcher indoors to give the air a fresh, sweet smell. To dry lavender, tie one-inch bundles together with string or elastic bands, and hang upside down until dry. You may want to place a clean cloth or large bowl beneath them to catch the flowers that fall.

Using Lavender

Anxiety- and Depression-Alleviating Tea

In a recent study comparing the effects of a medication for depression to drinking tea made from lavender flowers, scientists found that the lavender was slightly more effective than the antidepressant drugs. They concluded that lavender might be used as an adjunct to antidepressants or on its own to assist with symptoms of depression.[1] Study participants drank two cups of a lavender infusion daily.

To make lavender tea, add two teaspoons of dried flowers to boiled water, and let sit for 10 minutes. Strain and drink. Of course, never discontinue any medications without consulting your physician.

Insomnia Remedy

Due to its relaxing and antianxiety compounds, lavender is an excellent insomnia remedy. British hospitals have reportedly used lavender essential oil in patients' baths or sprinkled onto bedclothes to help them sleep. To use in a bath, sprinkle five to ten drops of lavender essential oil into the water as the tub fills. Alternatively, place a heaping tablespoon of dried lavender flowers in cheesecloth, tie into a bundle, and allow the herb to infuse in the bathwater while soaking.

Easy and Effective Insect Repellent

In a study comparing the effects of lavender essential oil to DEET-based tick repellents, the lavender showed results comparable to those of the DEET sprays. At a 5 percent concentration, the insect-repellent results of the lavender oil lasted for forty minutes; at a 10 percent or higher concentration, the results lasted for two hours.[2] Add ten to twenty drops of lavender essential oil to your favorite unscented cream, and apply before heading outdoors. Better yet, make your own Skin-Soothing Lavender Body Lotion (see recipe on page 108).

PMS Relief

A new study published in the journal *BioPsychoSocial Medicine* found that inhaling the scent of lavender for ten minutes had a significant effect on the nervous system of women suffering from premenstrual symptoms.[3] It especially decreased feelings of depression and confusion. You can place a few drops of lavender essential oil on a handkerchief and inhale periodically, make a tea infusion of the dried flowers as above, or deeply inhale the scent of a plant growing indoors or outdoors to alleviate PMS-related mood symptoms.

RECIPE

Skin-Soothing Lavender Body Lotion

It's easier than you think to make your own natural body lotion. Most of the ingredients can be found in your local health-food store. In place of the water in the recipe below, you can use an infusion made from one tablespoon of lavender flowers in 1 cup of water, infused for 10 to 20 minutes and then strained. If you are using a lavender infusion, you can omit the lavender essential oil if you prefer.

Makes about 2 cups.

¾ cup sweet almond oil
2 tablespoons shaved beeswax
30 drops lavender essential oil
1 cup water

Pour the oil into a small saucepan, add the beeswax, and heat the mixture over low to medium heat until the beeswax melts. Remove from the heat immediately. Allow to cool for a minute or two, but not longer, as the beeswax will begin to harden. Stir in the lavender essential oil.

Pour the water into a blender, cover, and begin blending it on high speed. With the blender running, slowly pour the beeswax mixture through the hole in the blender lid. The mixture will begin to thicken after about three-quarters of the beeswax has been incorporated.

Once all the beeswax has been blended, immediately pour the lotion into one 16-ounce glass jar or two 8-ounce glass jars. The lotion lasts about 6 months and is best kept in the fridge, since it contains no artificial preservatives.

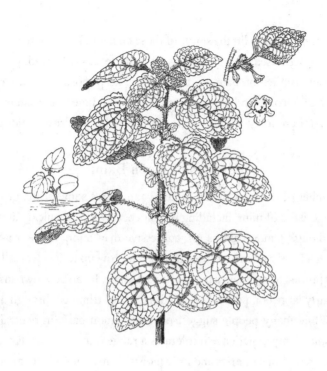

17. Lemon Balm

Melissa officinalis

Few people grow or use lemon balm, but if they knew about its impressive array of healing effects, this lovely, fragrant, and versatile plant would be popping up in gardens and kitchens everywhere.

A Brief History of Lemon Balm

Lemon balm was used as far back as the Middle Ages to improve sleep, reduce anxiety and stress, and relieve pain. In earlier times, lemon balm was steeped in wine and drunk to treat venomous bites and stings, to heal wounds, and to lift the spirits of those taking it. Like valerian, lemon balm has been used over the ages as a natural sedative. Nowadays, many gardeners rub lemon balm on their skin to keep mosquitoes at bay, although I'd recommend doing a patch test on your inner wrist and waiting twenty-four to forty-eight hours to check whether you're allergic.

Growing Lemon Balm

A member of the mint family, lemon balm shares some of the growing characteristics of mint, including its tendency to spread quickly and easily, although lemon balm is less aggressive than mint. While it usually reaches a height of two or three feet, it can grow up to five feet tall. It is easily pruned to maintain a more compact shape. It can be grown indoors in a fairly large pot, particularly if it is regularly trimmed through use.

While many people suggest planting lemon balm in neutral (7.0 pH) soil, in my experience it tolerates a range of conditions. Even in a climate with hot summers and little moisture, my lemon balm plant still thrives. It grows best, however, when watered weekly and planted in a location that is sunny but also gets some afternoon shade. It's easy to grow from seed or from a cutting of an existing plant placed in water, which should be changed daily. Once the plant has started to root, it can be planted in soil.

Lemon balm's botanical name is derived from the Greek *melissa*, which means "honeybee." Indeed, bees love it, and it's a great plant to grow organically in your garden to assist in restoring bee colonies, which have been decimated by pesticides and other environmental factors recently. Planting lemon balm near squash plants helps ensure pollination of the squash flowers.

Harvesting Lemon Balm

You can harvest the leaves and stems of lemon balm anytime, although I suggest waiting until a new plant has at least a few stems. The leaves are lovely when minced and added to green salads, fruit salads, or your favorite salsa. Because of the slight lemony scent, the leaves are also a great addition to fish, seafood, or poultry dishes.

The leaves and stems can also be used to make a mellow, relaxing tea by adding about one teaspoon of dried or one tablespoon of fresh lemon balm per cup of water and letting it steep for at least ten minutes.

Dry lemon balm by cutting about two-thirds of the way down the stems, tying them in bundles, and hanging them upside down. Store the dried lemon balm in a sealed glass jar.

Using Lemon Balm

Sedatives and thyroid medications may interact with lemon balm, so consult your physician prior to using lemon balm if you are taking either of these medications.

Herpes Virus Inhibitor

In a study published in the journal *Natural Products Research*, scientists found that lemon balm was highly effective against the herpes simplex virus.[1] This virus is responsible for the sexually transmitted disease herpes and for cold sores on the lips. Viruses must multiply in the body to survive. Lemon balm was shown to inhibit the ability of the herpes simplex virus to multiply by up to 60 percent. Other studies have shown the effectiveness of lemon balm ointment applied to herpes lesions and lip sores.[2]

HIV Inhibitor

A study reported in the medical journal *Retrovirology* found that lemon balm even showed activity against the human immunodeficiency virus (HIV). Scientists reported that lemon balm quickly and effectively slowed the entry of the virus into the cells.[3]

Headache Eliminator

Norman G. Bissett, who was professor of pharmacy at King's College London and the author of *Herbal Drugs and Phytopharmaceuticals*, recommended using lemon balm tea to treat headaches. Add one to two teaspoons of dried lemon balm to one cup of boiled water. Let the tea steep until it cools. Strain. Drink three cups daily whenever you're suffering from a headache.

Chronic Fatigue Syndrome Manager

My more than twenty years of clinical experience has shown that the antiviral herb lemon balm is a helpful treatment for chronic fatigue syndrome. Make a tea with one to two teaspoons of dried lemon balm per cup of boiled water. Drink a cup or two three times daily.

Insomnia Reducer

In a study of people with minor sleep problems, lemon balm combined with valerian was found to improve sleep quality in 81 percent of the participants.[4]

Healthy Thyroid Supporter

Anti-inflammatory herbs such as lemon balm are often recommended for relieving the inflammation associated with many thyroid conditions. Use thirty drops of tincture three times daily, or drink three cups of tea three times daily to support thyroid function.

RECIPES

Lemon Balm Tincture

This is the perfect at-home remedy to take during cold and flu season to prevent or treat viruses or cold sores.

Large bundle (2 to 3 cups) of fresh lemon balm, washed
One 750-ml bottle of vodka

Coarsely chop the leaves and stems of the lemon balm, and put it in a 16-ounce mason jar until it is about three-quarters full. Pour just enough of the vodka into the mason jar to completely submerge the lemon balm. Cover. Leave the jar in a cool, dark place for at least 4 weeks, shaking it once or twice daily, then strain out the plant matter. Store the tincture in a sealed jar for up to a year.

Take half a teaspoon of the tincture up to three times a day as necessary, or dab onto cold sores with a cotton swab.

Lemon Balm Vinegar

Use in place of plain vinegar in salad dressings or other recipes.
Makes 1 quart.

Large bundle (2 to 3 cups) of fresh lemon balm, washed
1 quart apple cider vinegar

Coarsely chop the lemon balm leaves and stems. Fill a 32-ounce mason jar about three-quarters full with the lemon balm. Add apple cider vinegar until all the lemon balm is submerged. Cover with a lid, and leave the jar in a cool, dark place for 2 to 4 weeks. Strain, and store in a sealed glass jar.

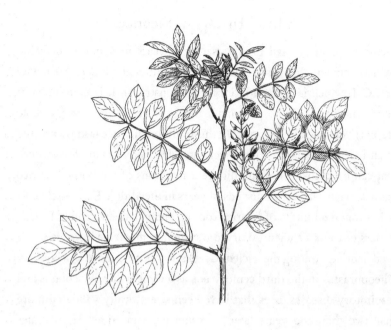

18. Licorice

Glycyrrhiza glabra

If I were stranded on a desert island and could only take one herb with me, it would be licorice. Licorice root is one of my favorite herbs, not only because it tastes like the candy that bears its name, or because it is one of the most profoundly healing herbs, but because it was one of the first herbs I used, and I believe that this wonderful healer played a significant role in restoring my health.

A Brief History of Licorice

Licorice has been used for thousands of years in Chinese medicine (which, incidentally, is not the same as Traditional Chinese Medicine, or TCM, which is a much more recent construct). It is mentioned in one of the classic Chinese medicine texts, the *Pen Ts'ao Ching* (Classic Herbal) published in 3000 BCE. In this tradition, licorice is known as the great harmonizer, which is a lovely and descriptive name for an herb that can harmonize so many different functions of the body. Licorice has also been used for thousands of years in the Middle East. Archaeologists found a bundle of licorice root in Tutankhamen's tomb. Practitioners of India's ancient Ayurvedic system of medicine have also long used licorice. Among the ancient Greeks, it was mentioned in a book by Theophrastus in the third century BCE as a remedy for dry coughs and respiratory diseases, uses that have been scientifically validated more than two thousand years later.[1] Around the same time, Hippocrates used the herb to treat coughs, asthma, and respiratory complaints. Hildegard von Bingen, a medieval German nun and herbalist, recommended licorice root for stomach and heart problems. Native Americans have also used licorice medicinally for many years, primarily as a tea, a laxative, and a remedy for coughs and earaches.[2] The Eclectic physicians of the nineteenth century in North America used licorice for bronchial and urinary tract problems, coughs, and colds. These physicians were the forerunners of traditional naturopathy, an approach that has unfortunately been marginalized in favor of a more medicalized approach to naturopathy.

Growing Licorice

Licorice loves dry, stony soil in full sun. You'll need to obtain a live rootstock or a live plant to grow it. Over time, this perennial plant will grow to approximately five feet tall. Wait until the shrub is quite mature before harvesting any of its roots.

Harvesting Licorice

When harvesting licorice root, remove outer roots only; don't dig too close to the rootstock, or you risk killing the plant. You can also use the outer bark from the stems, which have many of the same properties and the same delicious taste as the root. Finely chop the bark or roots, and dry in a 200°F oven until the roots are crisp but not brown. The fresh or dried root can be made into a decoction or tincture for medicinal use.

Using Licorice

Licorice is one of a relatively small group of herbs known as adaptogens. Adaptogens have the ability to improve overall body health, regulate body functions as needed, and give the body a boost to help it cope with physical, mental, or emotional stress of just about any kind. In other words, adaptogens help the body adapt (hence the name) to just about any stress it encounters.

Because it is such a powerful herb, however, licorice can have harmful side effects if misused, so it is important to use it with care. Individuals with high blood pressure or kidney failure, as well as people taking heart medication, should avoid licorice. It should not be used in large quantities or for periods longer than a few weeks without the guidance of a qualified herbalist or medical practitioner.

Adrenal Insufficiency Tonic

The adrenal glands, the body's primary glands that deal with stress, two small triangular glands that sit atop the kidneys, are vulnerable to stress from the pressures we face in our fast-paced modern world. The "adrenaline rush" many people get from driving themselves hard to excel or from extreme sports may seem great at the time, but over longer periods it can wear down the adrenal glands, causing a whole host of physical ailments, such as fatigue, poor digestion, sleep disorders, reduced immune system functioning, and elevated blood sugar levels.

Licorice is one of the best herbs to restore the body's hypothalamus-pituitary-adrenal axis (the HPA axis), a part of the endocrine system, which regulates the flow of adrenal outputs.

Immune System Regulator

Unlike drugs that can only either stimulate or reduce the function of an organ or organ system, licorice can both increase *and* decrease outputs of the body to bring about balance, depending on what is needed. This makes the herb a valuable choice for autoimmune disorders, in which an overactive immune system attacks the body's own tissues, including rheumatoid arthritis, lupus, and the skin condition known as scleroderma.

Anti-inflammatory Antidote

Increasing amounts of research link inflammation to over one hundred health conditions, including arthritis, cancer, diabetes, heart disease, and obesity. In a study in the medical journal *Natural Product Communications*, scientists compared the anti-inflammatory capabilities of several herbs to those of ibuprofen (Advil or Motrin). Licorice proved even more effective than ibuprofen[3] without the many serious side effects, such as liver damage.

Anticancer Medicine

Preliminary research in the medical journal *Fitoterapia* found that the compound glabridin, found in licorice root, was able to stop the ability of genes for liver cancer from turning on.[4] Other compounds in licorice demonstrate potential effectiveness against cancer of the digestive tract.[5] In breast cancer, the cancer's own stem cells are believed to cause metastasis (cancer spreading to other parts of the body) and recurrence of cancer. In the journal *Molecular Carcinogenesis*, scientists found that glabridin could inhibit cancer stem cells from spreading or causing the recurrence of breast cancer. The scientists conducting the study conclude that licorice root may be "a potential treatment strategy" and a way to "enhance the effectiveness of breast cancer therapy."[6]

Tooth Decay Preventer

Licorice root contains at least two compounds helpful in the prevention of tooth decay: the antibacterial compound glycyrrhizin and the potent decay-preventive compound known as indole.[7]

Chronic Fatigue Syndrome Solution

The Epstein-Barr virus has been found to be one of the many causal factors for chronic fatigue syndrome, or myalgic encephalomyelitis. Long-lasting and severe fatigue is only one of the symptoms of this serious, frequently disabling condition; others include severe muscle weakness and wasting, balance issues, digestive problems, bodily pain, and joint pain. Chronic fatigue syndrome has also been linked to an impaired blood-brain barrier, inflammation, liver impairment, adrenal gland weakness, stress, and other infections. Licorice root could be one of the most important herbs to treat this condition because of its adaptogenic properties. Research in the cancer journal *Oncotarget* found that the compounds quercetin and isoliquiritigenin in licorice showed activity against the Epstein-Barr virus implicated in chronic fatigue syndrome.[8]

Intestinal Health Booster

Licorice root reduces inflammation in the intestines and helps eliminate waste. Its role in protecting and healing damaged mucous membranes in the intestinal tract has been confirmed by hundreds of studies.[9] It also acts as a gentle laxative.

RECIPES

Anti-stress Tea

A cup of licorice tea can give you a boost when you are experiencing emotional or physical stress. Follow the instructions for a decoction on page 12.

Herbal Honey Ulcer Healer

3 tablespoons dried licorice, powdered
3 tablespoons dried marshmallow root, powdered
3–5 tablespoons unpasteurized honey

Combine all ingredients in a food processor until blended. Use only as much honey as needed to obtain a paste. Take one teaspoon three times daily to help soothe ulcers.

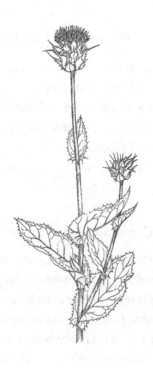

19. Milk Thistle

Silybum marianum

If you've ever pulled weeds from your garden, you're probably familiar with milk thistle. And attempts to remove it may not have gone so well because of its prickly stems and burrs that stick to clothing. Despite its outwardly pesky nature, milk thistle is one of the most powerful liver medicines available. While not a particularly attractive plant, and certainly not one you'd want to include in flower bouquets, milk thistle more than compensates for its less-than-appealing looks with therapeutic benefits.

A Brief History of Milk Thistle

Milk thistle has been used medicinally for over two thousand years. Dioscorides used it to treat snake bites. In the seventeenth century, the British herbalist Nicholas Culpeper was using milk thistle to treat jaundice, a yellowing of the skin and eyes that is a sign of liver dysfunction. The Eclectic physicians of nineteenth-century North America used the herb to treat liver conditions, varicose veins, menstrual disorders, and kidney problems.[1]

Growing Milk Thistle

Milk thistle may already grow in your garden, although it is probably not a plant you tend to pay attention to except to remove it. It is considered a biennial plant in warmer climates and an annual in colder ones. It can grow as tall as four to six feet and develops purple flowers in the summer when it matures. The seeds are the medicinal part of the plant. Each seed head produces between 100 and 190 seeds, which helps explain the plant's proliferation in fields and gardens across North America and Europe.[2] The seeds are mature when they've turned dark brown to black.

Considering its ability to thrive in wastelands, it is no surprise that the plant has no special soil requirements. It prefers full sunlight and minimal water.

Harvesting Milk Thistle

Wear thick gloves when working with this herb or harvesting its seeds.

Using Milk Thistle

Don't be fooled by milk thistle's modest history or unattractive appearance; this herb is potent medicine. More than one hundred studies have demonstrated milk thistle's effectiveness in detoxifying and strengthening the liver. It contains a compound called silymarin that protects the liver against cellular damage while also stimulating regeneration of

liver cells. Milk thistle also prevents the depletion of the nutrient gluta-
thione, which is essential for liver detoxification. And since the liver is
involved in over five hundred bodily functions, these properties make
milk thistle an important aid to overall health.

Unlike other liver herbs, milk thistle is best taken as a capsule or
as an alcohol extract. Because the substances silymarin and silybin are
not particularly water soluble, a tea made from the plant won't have
sufficient healing properties. Instead, take one teaspoon of the alcohol
extract three times daily (unless you have ever been an alcoholic) to
reap the medicinal benefits of milk thistle.

Liver Protector

By now you may have heard that over-the-counter painkillers like
acetaminophen (Tylenol) can cause liver damage. Research shows that
the use of milk thistle can help protect the liver from damage by these
drugs.[3]

Anticancer Agent

Numerous studies show that the compound silymarin found in
milk thistle seeds works on cancer in multiple ways: (1) it acts as an
antioxidant to eliminate cancer-causing free radicals; (2) it stabilizes
cellular membranes so that they are less vulnerable to damage; (3) it
stimulates detoxification pathways in the liver to help the body eliminate cancer-causing toxins; (4) it promotes liver tissue regeneration;
(5) it inhibits the growth of some cancer cell lines; (6) it acts directly on
some cancer cell lines to destroy them; and (7) it may increase the efficacy of some chemotherapy drugs.[4] Silybin is another compound found
in milk thistle that is believed to protect the genetic material within the
liver cells while reducing the occurrence of liver cancer.[5]

Liver Restorer Extraordinaire

Silymarin stimulates liver cell regeneration after the liver has been
damaged. It is a powerful liver tonic and helps alleviate indigestion,

which can be a sign that the liver is struggling to digest fats in the diet. Milk thistle is useful in the treatment of jaundice, cirrhosis, hepatitis, and liver poisoning.[6]

Milk Secretion Increaser

If you're nursing and finding that your milk is running dry, milk thistle can be used to increase milk secretion.[7]

Diabetes Preventer

Research reported in the medical journal *Diabetes, Metabolic Syndrome, and Obesity* found that an extract of milk thistle improved numerous markers of the conditions for which the journal is named, including reducing triglycerides, LDL cholesterol (often considered the harmful one), and blood sugar levels.[8] Interestingly, the herb worked even when statin drugs used to lower cholesterol were not tolerated.

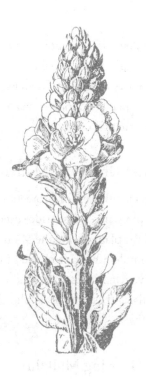

20. Mullein

Verbascum thapsus

Thanks to its soft and downy leaves, this plant is hard to miss, and that's a good thing. Because I live in a semiarid desert, wildfires are a threat every spring and summer. A carelessly discarded cigarette butt or an irresponsible bonfire in an ill-chosen setting can cause a single spark to travel along the root system of the forest floor and initiate a wildfire that can easily flare out of control. When that happens, the air thickens with smoke, causing difficulty breathing and the aggravation of respiratory conditions like asthma, COPD, and emphysema.

The velvety leaves of mullein offer a natural remedy for lung irritation caused by smoke. Interestingly, mullein (whose name rhymes with *sullen*) grows well in the hot, dry conditions of areas prone to wildfire, so I regularly seek out the tall plant to obtain its velvety leaves as a natural remedy against the lung irritation of smoke.

A Brief History of Mullein

Mullein was used in ancient cultures for protection against evil spirits. The first-century Greek physician Dioscorides used mullein to treat diarrhea. The French used the plant during the Middle Ages to treat boils on horses' necks. After mullein was introduced to North America by early settlers, many Native Americans quickly adopted the plant for use against coughs, bronchitis, and asthma — applications that research is now confirming as effective.

Growing Mullein

While mullein grows well in hot, dry conditions, it is also found in many other settings. It grows a tall, rod-like stem from which velvety leaves radiate. I've never planted mullein from seed or seedling, since it grows wild in my area. The plant grows up to five feet tall and yields small yellow flowers on the top of the stalk. It prefers dry, sandy, or somewhat rocky soil with good drainage and minimal water. If starting seeds indoors, wait until after the first frost to plant seedlings outside. Mullein can also be planted directly outdoors. Because of its size, it is not really suitable for growing indoors, but it could be grown in large pots outdoors.

Harvesting Mullein

To harvest mullein, I simply cut the base of the stalk and hang the whole plant upside down to dry in a clean, warm location. Once it has dried, I pull off the leaves and bag them. Some people pull the leaves off the stalk while they are still fresh, lay them out on baking sheets, and dry them in the oven on the lowest setting, but I don't recommend this option, as I feel the heat may destroy some of the medicinal compounds.

Using Mullein

Use one to two teaspoons of dried herb per cup of water to make infusions. Drink one cup of tea three times a day. You can also make a tincture from the fresh leaves. Take a quarter teaspoon to one teaspoon of tincture three times a day.

Allergy Assistance

Taken orally in tea or alcohol extract, mullein leaf helps to protect mucous membranes, thereby preventing them from triggering allergic reactions. It works when taken just prior to, during, or immediately after an allergic exposure. Of course, if you suffer from severe allergies and are at risk of an anaphylactic or other serious reaction, you should seek immediate medical attention.

Infection Fighter

In laboratory tests, researchers found that a mullein extract was effective against two harmful bacterial strains, *E. coli* and *Staphylococcus aureus*.[1]

Asthma Antidote

When taken daily, mullein can help relieve asthma and its symptoms, such as coughing and difficulty breathing. Mullein has also shown effectiveness for other respiratory conditions, such as coughs, whooping cough, and emphysema.

Mucous Membrane Soother

The leaves and flowers of the mullein plant lessen inflammation and pain in the mucous membranes, including those in the nasal lining, throat, lungs, and bronchial tubes.

Sexually Transmitted Disease Aid

New research published in the medical journal *Infectious Disorders Drug Targets* explored the use of mullein as an alternative to the potentially carcinogenic drug metronidazole in the treatment of trichomoniasis, a sexually transmitted infection caused by the parasite *Trichomonas vaginalis*. With the highest doses of mullein tested, over 86 percent of the parasites were destroyed, compared to only 2.9 percent in the control populations. These results suggest that mullein may be a good treatment option for this sexually transmitted disease.[2]

Tuberculosis Treatment

Research reported in the journal *Evidence-Based Complementary and Alternative Medicine* found that mullein is rich in compounds that seem to be particularly effective at attacking a group of bacteria known as mycobacteria, which are implicated in tuberculosis and other serious conditions.[3]

Worm Warrior

Mullein is used as a natural worm-killing medicine among some tribes in the Malakand region of Pakistan. A study of its effectiveness for this purpose, published in the online medical journal *BMC Complementary and Alternative Medicine*, found that mullein extract was more effective than the common worm medicine albendazole.[4]

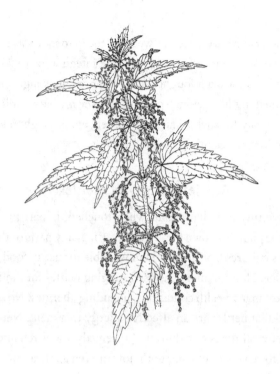

21. Nettles

Urtica dioica

Most people remember their first encounter with the aptly named stinging nettle. Mine came after my husband, Curtis, had completely torn up the front lawn of our first home. He told me that he wanted to create a beautiful garden for me. Over a period of weeks, he replaced the grass with rock paths and stone decorative features and planted a stunning garden, with over forty rose bushes and dozens of other strikingly beautiful plants. A smile crept across my face, and a sense of peace came over me each time I came home to this stunning beauty.

Sometime afterward, we were out weeding the garden. I was too lazy to get my gloves and grabbed a weed with the intention of yanking it out bare-handed, but the plant fought back with an instant stinging sensation that felt something like getting splinters all over my hand. Still, it was a small price to pay for such a stunning garden, and it taught me to make the minor effort to wear gloves while weeding.

A Brief History of Nettles

Nettles have tiny little hairs that, when touched, impart the stinging sensation the plant is known for. They grow in many parts of the world, and various cultures have found them valuable for use in food, textiles, and medicine. Native Americans used stinging nettles for thousands of years to treat many health conditions, including allergies. Now, science has proved that nettles are an effective allergy treatment. Nettles were used in medieval times as a diuretic (to remedy water retention in the body) and to relieve joint pain, both now proven applications.

I recently discovered that there is an annual nettle-eating competition in the United Kingdom — an interesting, albeit rather painful, tradition. It's probably unnecessary to mention it, but I don't recommend following this lead by eating raw nettles.

Growing Nettles

Nettles germinate readily in the spring, and indeed you may already be growing them in damp and shady parts of your garden.

Harvesting Nettles

Wear gloves while planting seedlings or harvesting these herbs. If you're stung, apply freshly pulverized plantain leaves to the area to relieve the stinging sensation. It takes only about thirty seconds of cooking to eliminate the sting. The leaves can be added to soups and stews, sautéed like spinach or other green leafy vegetables, or dried for use in teas. However, if you want to skip the nettle-picking experience, they are also readily available for purchase in dried form, as tinctures, and in drop or capsule form. Medicinally, fresh nettles are far superior to dried ones, so it is worth donning a pair of gloves to harvest this healing plant. Avoid the topical use of nettles on open wounds, and do not ingest them during pregnancy.

Using Nettles

Allergy Antidote

Modern research supports the traditional Native American use of nettles to alleviate allergies. In a study published in the medical journal *Phytotherapy Research*, researchers at the company HerbalScience Group found that nettles worked on multiple levels to significantly reduce inflammation linked to allergies.[1] Unlike many pharmaceutical antiallergy medications, nettles do not cause heart problems or drowsiness.

Bone Builder

Nettles are a nutritional powerhouse, containing an abundance of calcium in a form that is more readily absorbed into the body than that found in dairy products.

Diabetes Therapy

Research published in the journal *Neuroscience Letters* found that nettles showed tremendous potential for alleviating many of the health problems linked to diabetes, including reducing blood sugar levels, reducing the symptom of excessive thirst, facilitating weight management, regulating insulin levels, reducing neuropathic pain, and even improving memory and cognition.[2]

Pain Reliever

Nettles have been shown to interfere with pain signals transmitted through the nervous system, thereby reducing pain from arthritis, gout, other types of joint problems, muscle aches, tendinitis, sprains, and strains. To obtain the effect, however, you'll need to expose the painful area to stings by brushing it with the fine nettle hairs. The stinging sensation is temporary and ultimately helps reduce the original pain.[3] Some studies suggest that taking a nettle extract internally can help reduce the pain of osteoarthritis and thus enable sufferers to reduce their doses of anti-inflammatory pharmaceutical drugs.[4]

Prostate Treatment

Nettles have been found to be superior to the drug finasteride in the treatment of the prostate condition known as benign prostatic hyperplasia (BPH), a condition in which the prostate becomes enlarged and presses on the urethra (the tube that carries urine from the bladder), thereby reducing urine flow and causing incomplete emptying of the bladder. Although the effect is not completely understood, the researchers are clear that nettles work as effectively as the common drug used to treat this condition.[5]

Sinus Solution

In a recent double-blind study, the leaves of the stinging nettle were investigated for their ability to relieve allergic rhinitis. Participants taking nettles had noticeably higher relief from symptoms than those taking the placebo.[6]

RECIPE

Spring Nettle and Tarragon Soup

My friend Dylan W. Foss, an executive chef, is well known for his delicious soups, among many other foods he prepares. He agreed to share one of his famous soup recipes with me. It's the perfect way to enjoy calcium-rich, allergy-fighting nettles, particularly in the springtime, when they first start rearing their heads in gardens.

Serves 4 to 6.

2 tablespoons extra-virgin olive oil
3 stalks celery, sliced
1 large onion, chopped
5 cloves garlic, diced
2 tablespoons white wine
4 cups water
¼ cup fresh tarragon, loosely packed
2 cups fresh nettle leaves, loosely packed
Salt to taste
Apple cider vinegar to taste

In a medium saucepan, heat the oil until it's warm but not smoking. Add the celery, onion, and garlic, and sauté until the vegetables are translucent. Add the wine, and boil to reduce the liquid. Add the water, and bring the broth to a boil again. Add the tarragon and nettles, and cook until tender, 2 to 4 minutes. Purée the soup in a blender or using an immersion blender, and season with salt and apple cider vinegar. Serve immediately.

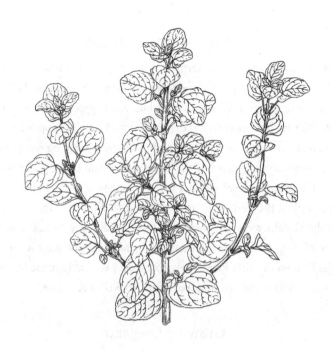

22. Oregano

Origanum vulgare

I love Greek food: salads, tzatziki (yogurt dip), and other specialties. Garlic and oregano are among the signature flavors of this cuisine. While many people tend to think of herbs in distinct categories of use, such as culinary or medicinal, oregano proves that there is significant crossover between them. Not only is oregano a robust flavor addition to salads, vegetables, poultry, and meat dishes, but it is also a potent natural medicine, proving the truth of the old adage "Food is the best medicine."

A Brief History of Oregano

It will probably come as no surprise that oregano was first used by the Greeks. Indeed, the ancient Greeks believed that the goddess Aphrodite invented oregano to make the lives of humans happier. I can only speak for one human, but oregano has definitely made my life happier. The ancient Greeks crowned newlyweds with wreaths containing oregano and placed sprigs on the graves of the deceased to help bring peace to their spirits. These ancients were also aware of oregano's medicinal properties and prescribed the herb regularly for the treatment of many afflictions. After the Greeks were conquered by the Romans, the Romans adopted the use of oregano in their diet and medicine, disseminating it throughout the Roman Empire. From there, oregano eventually made its way to China and, within the last hundred years, to North America.[1]

Growing Oregano

Provided with fertile, well-drained soil and full sun, oregano will grow in a wide variety of places. It can be grown from seed indoors and planted outdoors after the last frost, or it can be kept indoors in a pot. Space plants about twelve inches apart. Oregano tends to start slowly and grow faster as it receives more warmth. As a result, it is important to keep young plants well weeded, since weeds can quickly overtake them. Because many other plants are sold as oregano, look for the Latin name *Origanum vulgare*.

Harvesting Oregano

For cooking, harvest only the leaves. Both the leaves and the stems can be used in the making of natural medicines. To dry, collect the oregano stems (with leaves intact) together, tie in bundles up to an inch thick, and hang upside down to dry. Store in an airtight container. Dried oregano retains its flavor and potency for up to six months.

Using Oregano

In addition to drying the herb, you can make oregano tinctures from the chopped leaves and stems to use whenever you feel a virus coming on. Taking oregano at the first sign of a sore throat or fever can often prevent illness, so I always keep this herb handy.

Infection Fighter

Oregano is a powerfully antiseptic plant, thanks to the compounds known as carvacrol and rosmarinic acid. As opposed to antibiotic drugs, which act only against bacteria, these compounds work against bacteria, viruses, fungi, and even parasites like worms, making oregano a well-rounded antiseptic for your natural medicine cabinet. Research reported in the journal *Microbial Ecology in Health and Disease* showcased oregano's effectiveness against *Klebsiella oxytoca* and *Klebsiella pneumoniae*.[2] These bacteria can infect the skin, wounds, throat, gastrointestinal tract, urinary tract, and particularly the lungs.[3] Research published in the journal *Frontiers in Microbiology* showcased the effectiveness of oregano against antibiotic-resistant strep infections, particularly strep throat.[4] This study used essential oil, which is a particularly potent extract of the oil components of the plant. It takes many pounds of oregano to extract a small amount of oil, so for this purpose you're better off purchasing an undiluted bottle of oregano oil from your local health-food store or making your own alcohol-based tincture of oregano.

Super Antioxidant

Dozens of sources show that oregano has demonstrated significant antioxidant activity, making it effective in preventing or alleviating many health conditions caused or aggravated by the presence of free radicals in the body.[5]

Glaucoma Preventer

Free radicals are involved in the eye condition glaucoma, which causes damage to the optic nerve and can result in vision loss or blindness. If glaucoma runs in your family or you have been diagnosed with the condition, it is best to incorporate plentiful amounts of antioxidants, and particularly oregano, in your diet.

Arthritis Antidote

Because of its anti-infectious and antioxidant properties, oregano can be helpful in the treatment of both rheumatoid and osteoarthritis. While infections have only been implicated in rheumatoid arthritis, both types of arthritis benefit from oregano's potent antioxidant activity.

Blood Pressure Balancer

According to the research of the renowned herbalist James Duke, oregano contains seven natural compounds that reduce high blood pressure, making it a great regular dietary addition for anyone suffering from the condition.[6]

Cancer Remedy

While oregano hasn't been studied extensively for use against cancer, preliminary studies published in the *Journal of Medicinal Food* showed that the compound 4-terpineol found in oregano was effective at inhibiting the spread of cancer.[7] In an article in the journal *Food and Chemical Toxicology*, researchers reported that oregano particularly targeted liver cancer cells to destroy them.[8]

Asthma Aid

According to James Duke, oregano contains four antiasthma compounds.[9] The oil or tincture should be ingested, not inhaled, when used for asthma. Actually, it is important not to breathe too deeply when using oregano with asthma, especially the essential oil, since the powerful aromatic compounds can initiate a cough reflex that can temporarily aggravate asthma.

Emphysema and Lung Infection Remedy

James Duke identified six compounds in oregano that help expel mucus from the lungs (expectorants), making the herb an excellent choice for treating emphysema or lung infections.[10] These expectorant compounds also work on mucus in the sinuses, so you might find oregano helpful in treating sinus infections as well. Use in the same way as for asthma (see above).

RECIPES

Greek-Style Quinoa

Quinoa is high in fiber and protein, making it an excellent food to help stabilize blood sugar levels (blood sugar fluctuations are an underlying factor in many serious health conditions) and maintain a healthy weight. You can make this salad ahead of time and refrigerate it for up to 3 days for a quick and easy meal when you're short on time.

Serves 2 to 4.

1 cup quinoa
1 ½ to 2 cups water
1 tablespoon fresh basil, chopped
1 tablespoon fresh oregano leaves, chopped
½ onion, diced
Juice of 1 lemon
½ teaspoon unrefined sea salt
1 tablespoon extra-virgin olive oil
1 red bell pepper, diced
½ cucumber, diced

Cook the quinoa in the water according to package instructions. Allow to cool. In a separate bowl, combine the basil, oregano, onion, lemon juice, salt, and olive oil. Set aside for 5 to 10 minutes. When the quinoa has cooled, add the pepper, cucumber, and lemon-onion mixture. Toss all the ingredients together. Eat immediately or refrigerate.

Super-Healing Greek Salad

I make Greek salad often, varying the ingredients slightly each time. This one is my favorite.

Serves 2 to 4.

Salad vegetables
    1 large cucumber, chopped
    3 medium tomatoes, chopped
    1 large red bell pepper, chopped
    ½ small purple onion, thinly sliced
    Handful of fresh mint, finely chopped

Dressing
    Juice of 2 lemons (about 6 tablespoons)
    1 cup extra-virgin olive oil
    1 teaspoon dried basil
    Small handful of fresh oregano leaves
    ½ teaspoon black pepper
    ½ teaspoon unrefined sea salt
    Dash of cayenne pepper

Place the cucumber, tomatoes, bell pepper, onion, and mint in a large bowl. Using a bowl and whisk, a small food processor, or a blender, thoroughly blend the lemon juice, olive oil, basil, oregano, pepper, salt, and cayenne. Pour the dressing over the salad vegetables, toss, and let sit for at least 30 minutes to allow the flavors to combine.

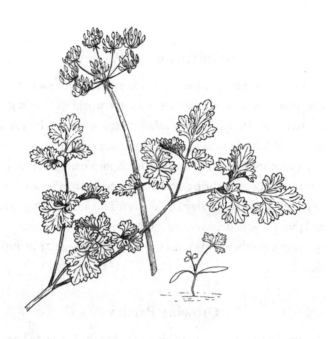

23. Parsley

Petroselinum sativum

While many people probably think of parsley as nothing more than a garnish served alongside their restaurant meals, this herb warrants greater inclusion in our diet and natural medicine cabinet. Not only is it packed with nutrients, but it also helps prevent diabetes, can prevent and treat kidney stones, and is a proven, all-natural anticancer remedy. It's definitely time to rethink this humble and overlooked herb. Parsley offers many health-boosting properties, is simple to grow, and makes a delicious addition to most meals.

A Brief History of Parsley

Native to southern Europe, parsley has been in use for more than two thousand years and is now grown around the world. According to the Roman statesman Pliny, "Not a salad or sauce should be presented without it."[1] While we tend to think of parsley primarily as a culinary herb, our ancestors thought of it primarily as medicine. They used parsley to treat gallstones, arthritis, and insect bites, and as an aphrodisiac. They also believed that parsley could absorb the intoxicating fumes of wine and thus prevent drunkenness.[2] Obviously that is not the case, but parsley has many other proven uses to warrant its regular inclusion in your diet.

Growing Parsley

Growing parsley is easy. You can choose either the flat-leafed or curly-leafed varieties, depending on your preference. Parsley is a biennial plant, which means that it grows for two years before you need to start new plants from seed. To give the plants a head start on spring, plant seeds indoors about ten to twelve weeks before the last frost in individual pots. It takes a while to germinate, so be patient. Keep the soil moist to prevent seedlings from drying out.[3] Set parsley plants outdoors, six to eight inches apart, approximately three to four weeks before the last frost. Parsley particularly likes to be planted near tomatoes, corn, or asparagus, but it is fairly tolerant and easy to grow. You can also plant parsley directly from seed or seed tape into your garden or grow it indoors on a windowsill or in a sunny spot. If you want fresh parsley throughout the winter, transplant an outdoor parsley plant into a pot, and keep it on your windowsill.

Harvesting Parsley

To harvest, wait until the leaf stems have three segments. After that, cut outer portions of the plant as needed. To dry parsley, tie one-inch bundles of stems together and hang upside down until dry. Once dry, store in an airtight jar. You can also chop or purée fresh parsley (stems included), mix it with olive oil, and freeze the mixture in ice-cube trays. Once the cubes are frozen, place them in a freezer bag for storage. Simply pop a cube into a soup, stew, or pasta dish, or thaw and use to make a fresh vinaigrette for your salads.

Using Parsley

Parsley is one of the most versatile herbs, making it easy to benefit from this herb's many health-promoting properties. Parsley leaves and stems can be finely chopped and added to soups, stews, salads, pasta dishes, fresh juices, and more.

Nutrition Booster

Parsley is high in many nutrients, including vitamins A and C, as well as the minerals iron and sulfur.

Anticancer Powerhouse

A new study in the *Journal of the Science of Food and Agriculture* found that parsley has potent anticancer properties. It acts as an antioxidant that destroys free radicals before they damage cells, protects DNA from damage that can lead to cancer or other diseases, and inhibits the proliferation and migration of cancer cells in the body.[4]

Diabetes Prevention

Research published in the *Journal of Nutrition* found that eating foods high in a naturally occurring nutrient known as myricetin can decrease the risk of developing type 2 diabetes by 26 percent.[5] Parsley is one of the best sources of myricetin, containing about 8 milligrams per 100 grams of parsley.[6] The study, known as the European Prospective Investigation into Cancer and Nutrition (Epic), was conducted in twenty-six study centers in eight European countries over several years. A subsequent study of 12,403 people with type 2 diabetes showed a strong link between consumption of flavonol (a natural compound found in parsley) and a significantly reduced incidence of the disease.[7]

Kidney Stone Preventer

Kidney stones — mineral crystals that lodge in the kidney or urinary tract — can be an excruciatingly painful complaint. One mineral commonly implicated in the formation of kidney stones is calcium oxalate. In a study published in *Urology Journal*, researchers found that ingesting parsley leaf and roots reduced the number of calcium oxalate deposits in animals. The researchers also found that ingesting parsley helped break down kidney stones in animals.[8]

RECIPES

Gluten-Free Tabbouleh Salad

Popular in Middle Eastern and Mediterranean countries, tabbouleh is traditionally made with bulgur wheat, but it gets an easy gluten-free twist and a nutrition boost when it's made with quinoa instead. This recipe is quick and easy to prepare, but the flavors deepen after it sits in the fridge for an hour or two, or even overnight.

Serves 4.

2 tomatoes, chopped
1 large bunch fresh parsley or 2 small bunches, finely chopped
1 clove garlic, minced
1 green onion, chopped
2 cups cooked quinoa
Juice of 3 lemons (about ½ cup)
2 tablespoons extra-virgin olive oil
½ teaspoon Celtic sea salt or Himalayan salt
Pinch of cayenne pepper

In a large bowl, combine the tomatoes, parsley, garlic, green onion, and quinoa. In a small bowl, whisk together the lemon juice, olive oil, salt, and cayenne. Pour the mixture over the salad, and toss to coat.

Store the tabbouleh in an airtight container in the refrigerator for up to 4 days. The flavors will mingle, making the salad taste even better.

Parsley Power Juice

This delicious and nutritious juice, drunk regularly, can help you benefit from the anticancer and antidiabetes properties of parsley. Wash but do not peel the vegetables or apple to retain as many nutrients as possible.

Makes approximately 1½ cups.

Large handful of parsley
6 carrots
1 cucumber
1 apple

Push all ingredients through a juicer, alternating the parsley with the vegetables and apple to avoid clogging your juicer. Drink immediately.

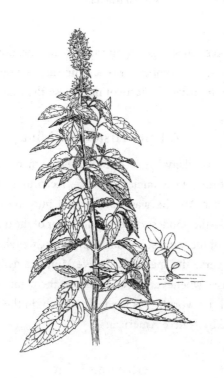

24. Peppermint

Mentha x piperita

For some people, the mention of mint conjures images of candy canes and chewing gum, but the many uses of fragrant, versatile, and easy-growing mint extend far beyond the candy counter. In the kitchen, mint makes an excellent addition to recipes and an uplifting tea. Among the easiest plants in the world to grow, aromatic mint is a lovely and low-maintenance garden perennial. The varieties peppermint and spearmint, longtime favorites in the medicine chest, are rich in antioxidants, and they can help freshen breath, relieve sinus congestion, alleviate indigestion and gastrointestinal concerns, improve breathing, treat gallstones, and combat viruses. Mint makes a delicious tea on its own and also improves the taste of many less-than-tasty herbal teas.

A Brief History of Mint

Although it very likely began even earlier, human use of peppermint has been recorded since ancient Greece. According to Greek legend, a nymph named Minthe was transformed into the mint plant when Persephone — the goddess of spring and later of the underworld — became jealous of the interest her husband, Pluto, was showing in Minthe. Unable to reverse the spell, Pluto gave Minthe a delightful scent that filled the senses whenever anyone trod on the plant. Varieties of mint grow around the world. It is used extensively in the Middle East and was also used by Native Americans.[1]

Growing Mint

The twenty-five types of mint include the well-known varieties such as peppermint and spearmint, as well as more exotic varieties, such as apple, orange, and chocolate mint. You don't need a green thumb to grow mint, although you may have one after harvesting it, thanks to its rich chlorophyll content. Often the problem with mint is not getting it to grow but restraining it: it grows thick underground stems that can spread throughout the garden and overtake neighboring plants. If you want to confine mint to one section of your garden, you may want to plant it in a container at least fifteen inches deep and then place the container in the soil. Mints also grow happily indoors in pots; just be sure to choose a fairly large pot to give the plant room to spread.

Mint prefers a cool, moist spot but can easily grow in full sun if watered regularly. Indoor potting soil provides sufficient nutrients for a few months. After that, fertilize mint plants using about half of the amount suggested on a package of organic fertilizer for indoor plants.[2]

Harvesting Mint

Pluck mint leaves off plants as needed, or snip sprigs about an inch above the soil. To dry mint, cut off sprigs an inch above the soil, wash, dry, tie the stems in one-inch bundles, and hang upside down in a dark, dry place. Once the leaves are dry, pull them off the stems and store them in an airtight container for up to a year.

Using Mint

Tasty Treat

When cooking, add chopped mint to vegetable dishes, rice bowls, fruit or vegetable salads, and soups (especially gazpacho). Mint is great with lamb dishes.

Breath Booster

Research shows that the rosmarinic acid contained in peppermint blocks inflammatory compounds called leukotrienes and encourages the body to make prostacyclins, which open the airway and improve breathing. Peppermint has also been shown to alleviate nasal congestion linked to colds and allergies; drinking peppermint tea works well for this purpose.[3]

Cold Killer

Dominion Herbal College in Burnaby, British Columbia, recommends a strong mint and elderflower tea to promote perspiration and fend off colds and flu. To make this traditional remedy, steep one tablespoon each of peppermint leaves and elderflowers (available from online herbal suppliers) in hot water. Drink a half to a full cup every thirty to forty-five minutes at the first sign of a cold or flu, until you start perspiring. Then take two tablespoons every hour or two until the fever breaks or the symptoms improve.[4]

Sinus Aid and Facial Spritzer

Peppermint relieves sinusitis.[5] If your sinuses feel congested, drink a cup of peppermint tea two to three times daily. You can also use peppermint tea as a facial spritzer, although you'll need to brew it regularly, as it won't last for more than a week if kept in the fridge. Alternatively, rub a drop or two of peppermint essential oil on your temples. (Be careful not to get it in your eyes, as it can burn.)

Tummy Tamer

Sip a cup of peppermint tea to alleviate nausea, vomiting, and digestive upset.[6]

Gallstone Savior

Thanks to the compound borneol, found in numerous varieties of mint, James Duke, botanist and author of *The Green Pharmacy*, recommends "stone tea" as an aid in the elimination of gallstones (along with any prescribed medical treatment). He suggests mixing as many different types of mint as you have available, but especially peppermint and spearmint, with a teaspoon of cardamom, brewing as tea, and drinking frequently.[7]

Herpes Helper

According to research by John Heinerman, a doctor of medical anthropology and author of *Healing Herbs and Spices*, peppermint is potent against viruses, making it a good choice in dealing with the herpes virus. The *Herpes simplex* virus causes cold sores and genital herpes. *Herpes zoster* is linked to chicken pox and shingles. Heinerman recommends two cups of hot peppermint tea daily to alleviate symptoms and shorten the duration of herpes outbreaks.[8] Once in the body, the herpes virus is always present, but it can remain dormant. Occasionally drinking peppermint tea can help reduce the chances of an outbreak.

Road Rage Reliever

Let's face it: most people occasionally experience road rage, anxiety, fatigue, or frustration while driving. Research by Bryan Raudenbush, an associate professor of psychology at Wheeling Jesuit University in Wheeling, West Virginia, may have the solution. He found that inhaling the scent of peppermint or cinnamon while driving a car decreased levels of frustration, anxiety, and fatigue. The scent of natural peppermint (not artificial fragrances) also increased alertness while driving. You can keep a sachet of dried peppermint in your car, use peppermint essential oil in an aromatherapy diffuser, or keep some freshly brewed peppermint tea in your travel mug to stay calm on the road.[9]

RECIPES

Mint Magic Tea

To make mint tea, use one teaspoon of dried mint per cup of hot water. Mint's natural oils are best extracted in hot, but not boiling, water. Let the tea steep for 10 minutes.

Peppermint Salt Body Scrub

Use this scrub to improve circulation and maintain healthy skin. Unrefined sea salt is full of skin-healing minerals, the essential oils eliminate harmful microbes and heal blemishes, and the olive oil moisturizes the skin. Note that essential oil is not the same as extract or fragrance oil. Choose an essential oil that is labeled "food grade" or "pharmaceutical grade."

Makes about ¾ cup.

2 tablespoons ground dried peppermint leaves or 20 drops
    peppermint essential oil

¼ cup extra-virgin olive oil
½ cup finely ground, unrefined sea salt

In a small bowl, mix the peppermint leaves or essential oil with the olive oil and sea salt. Pour into a jar to store. To use, massage the scrub into damp skin. Rinse and pat skin dry.

Natural Tooth Powder

Peppermint essential oil helps freshen breath, kill bacteria, and clear sinuses. Myrrh oil is highly antibacterial and antifungal. Baking soda restores a natural, slightly alkaline pH balance to the teeth and gums.
Makes ½ cup.

½ cup baking soda
10 drops peppermint essential oil
5 drops myrrh essential oil (optional)

Combine the ingredients in a small jar with a lid, cover, and shake well. Use a small amount on a damp toothbrush, as you would use toothpaste.

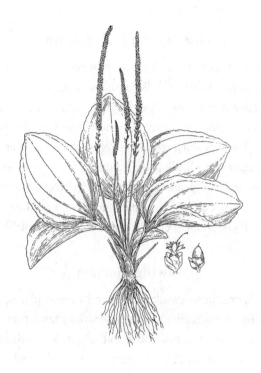

25. Plantain

Plantago major

A weed that you've probably trampled on more than a few times could help you butt out or transform your health. The North American wild herb plantain (which is not related to the banana-like plant found in the Caribbean) helps reduce cravings for cigarettes and is used in many commercial smoking-cessation products. But this use is just one of the myriad reasons to stop treading on this herb and start enjoying it instead.

A Brief History of Plantain

Plantain has been grown and used in Europe for centuries and was brought by Europeans to North America. Because it seemed to show up wherever they went, Native Americans called the plant "white man's foot" or "Englishman's foot." Another Native American name for the plant means "life medicine," and modern research suggests that it is an apt testament to the plant's impressive healing and health-giving properties. Both Native Americans and Europeans frequently carried plantain root with them for use on snake bites, a use that is still common today. Plantain has since established itself just about everywhere and is readily available.

Growing Plantain

Growing on lawns, in sidewalk cracks, and in wild places, plantain is regularly killed by grass aficionados in search of lawn perfection. You may be growing it right now without realizing it. While there are many different types of plantain, the varieties most often found in lawns are low-lying and have either a long, thin leaf or a short, broad leaf.

Harvesting Plantain

You can harvest fresh, young plantain leaves from unsprayed areas. You can also harvest the leaves anytime from early spring until the frost and hang them upside down to dry for use later as a tea.

Using Plantain

Fresh plantain leaves can be used in salads, steamed or sautéed like spinach, or made into a fresh herb tincture. Smokers trying to quit can fill a small spray bottle with the tincture and spritz it into the mouth to help quell the urge to smoke.

Nutrition and Overall Health Booster

Plantain is packed with nutrients, including beta carotene, calcium, vitamins C and K, and phytonutrients like allantoin, apigenin, aucubin, baicalein, oleanolic acid, sorbitol, and tannin.[1] Beta carotene boosts eyesight and helps fight cancer, calcium builds strong bones and is essential to a healthy nervous system, vitamin C helps fight cancer and reduces the effects of stress, and vitamin K is necessary for blood and blood-vessel health. Allantoin[2] and apigenin are potent natural anti-inflammatories, aucubin can heal damaged or injured nerves,[3] baicalein can aid in the repair of mitochondria (the cells' energy centers),[4] and oleanolic acid has antiviral and liver-protecting qualities.[5]

Smoking Cessation Aid

Plantain seems to create a natural aversion to cigarettes, thereby making it easier to leave them behind. It can be used in various forms: tea, tincture, or spray. For a tea, simply add one teaspoon of dried plantain to a cup of boiling water, steep for at least ten minutes, strain, then drink before you reach for a cigarette. Many people find that this eliminates the craving or that they don't want to smoke a whole cigarette. Plantain tincture or quit-smoking spray should be used according to the package directions, usually just prior to lighting up.

Respiratory Booster

Not only does plantain reduce cravings for cigarettes, but it is also used by natural health practitioners to reduce bronchial congestion, laryngitis, lung irritation and inflammation, and coughs. Multiple studies indicate that plantain has demonstrated abilities to heal bronchitis as well as upper-respiratory conditions.[6]

Cancer Answer

Research published in the *Journal of Ethnopharmacology* found that an extract of plantain strongly suppressed the growth of human cancer cells, suggesting that this herb could play an important role in addressing cancer naturally or in combination with chemotherapy or radiotherapy.[7] The scientists also believe that plantain may help prevent the damage to DNA normally caused by cancer cells.

General Health Tonic

Plantain has been used to relieve toothaches, ulcers, digestive complaints, gout, and kidney infections.

RECIPE

Smoking Cessation Tea

If you're trying to quit smoking, this tea can help. Simply drink some of this herbal tea when you feel the urge to smoke. You can add a touch of honey or the natural sweetener stevia if you prefer a sweeter tea. If you're still not wild about the taste of this herbal tea, you can also add one teaspoon of dried peppermint while brewing.

> 1 cup water
> 1 teaspoon dried plantain leaves or 1 tablespoon fresh plantain
>   leaves

In a small saucepan, boil the water. Stir in the plantain leaves, cover, and let the mixture steep for at least 10 minutes. Strain. Drink one to three cups daily for best results.

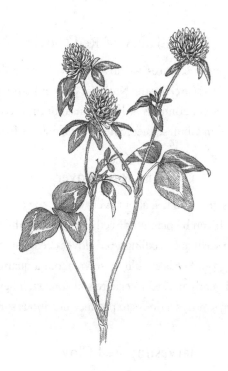

26. Red Clover

Trifolium pratense

As a child I would spend hours on the lawn looking for four-leaf clovers, lucky charms that would make my dreams come true. Although I occasionally found a four-leaf clover, and even one time a five-leaf clover, I can't say what role, if any, these had in shaping the life I currently lead. But if clover brings luck, one way it may do so is through its health-giving properties.

A Brief History of Red Clover

Thirty-three different cultures worldwide have used red clover as a cancer treatment.[1] Research by the National Cancer Institute (NCI) has verified that red clover contains at least four antitumor compounds. It has also been used in Chinese medicine to expel mucus from the lungs.

Growing Red Clover

Red clover grows on lawns just about everywhere, so you can easily cultivate your own. It can be planted directly in soil after the last frost has passed. Like most seeds and seedlings, red clover needs sufficient warmth and moisture to grow. Seeds should be sown about a quarter of an inch deep and the soil gently packed to ensure soil contact. They can also be germinated in trays or jars indoors to produce nutritious sprouts.

Harvesting Red Clover

The flowers can be plucked and dried or made into a tincture. When I lay out the flowers on a baking sheet, I find they air-dry quite quickly.

Using Red Clover

For therapeutic uses, mainly the flowers are used, in tinctures and teas. Both the flowers and the leaves can be added to salads. Red clover sprouts make an excellent addition to sandwiches or salads.

Breast Cancer Fighter

Red clover contains a natural compound known as formononetin that helps combat breast cancer. According to research published in the medical journal *Hormone and Metabolic Research*, formononetin helps prevent cancer cell migration and invasion of healthy cells so that the disease is less likely to spread.[2] This research is significant not only for the promise of healing breast cancer but also because it challenges earlier recommendations against the use of clover. Previously, the herb was assumed to have effects similar to those of estrogen drugs, and people suffering from estrogen-aggravated cancers were advised to avoid this herb altogether. The new findings are controversial, however, so you should draw your own conclusions.

Heart Disease Aid

Multiple studies show that red clover may help in the prevention and treatment of heart disease. One study found that red clover improved arterial elasticity,[3] while another, published in the *European Journal of Clinical Nutrition*, found that it reduced high levels of LDL (bad) cholesterol.[4] Although the importance of blood cholesterol levels is debated, excessive amounts can still contribute to heart disease.

Menopause Marvel

While there is controversy over whether red clover alleviates menopausal symptoms, the herb seems to help women whose symptoms are linked to estrogen imbalances, as opposed to progesterone or testosterone imbalances. Many health practitioners seem to believe that all the symptoms of menopause can be addressed by a single type of treatment, but in my experience women experience difficult menopausal symptoms for different reasons, depending on which hormones are implicated, and red clover can be effective for those who suffer from insufficient estrogen, especially those who experience hot flashes. Red clover contains natural estrogenic substances known as isoflavones that can help boost low levels of estrogen in the body. Isoflavones can also attach to estrogen receptor sites in the body to help reduce estrogen levels when necessary, since they are much gentler than human estrogen or estrogens found in the foods we eat. A typical dose is two to three cups of red clover tea daily.

Osteoporosis Answer

Research published in the medical journal *Evidence-Based Complementary and Alternative Medicine* found that the formononetin found in red clover helped prevent the development of osteoporosis in animals.[5]

RECIPE

Hormone-Balancing Tea

It's easy to benefit from red clover's natural hormone-balancing properties by enjoying this herbal tea on a daily basis. You can add a touch of honey or the natural sweetener stevia if you prefer a sweeter tea. If you're still not wild about the taste of this herbal tea, you can also add one teaspoon of dried peppermint while brewing.

> 1 cup water
> 1 teaspoon dried red clover flowers or 1 tablespoon fresh red
>   clover flowers

In a small saucepan, boil the water. Stir in the clover flowers, cover, and let the mixture steep for at least 10 minutes. Strain. Drink one to three cups daily for best results.

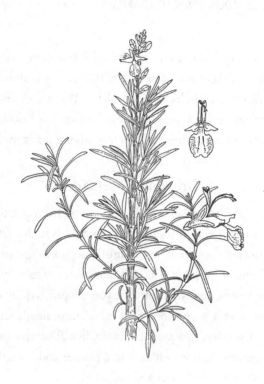

27. Rosemary

Rosmarinus officinalis

I keep a rosemary topiary in a pot at my front door and run my hands through its branches to send the delightful smell wafting through the air to enjoy its delightful aroma. Rosemary is a great seasoning for meat dishes, and now, with confirmation of its many health benefits, there are more reasons than ever to enjoy this fragrant herb.

A Brief History of Rosemary

The Latin name *Rosmarinus*, which means "dew of the sea," is probably linked to the plant's native region, the Mediterranean. In many cultures, rosemary has been associated with remembrance and memory. Rosemary sprigs have been laid as tributes on coffins and tombstones. In *Hamlet*, Ophelia tells Hamlet, "There's rosemary, that's for remembrance; pray, love, remember." In ancient Greece, students stuck rosemary sprigs in their hair when studying for exams.

Growing Rosemary

You can propagate rosemary by taking a cutting from an existing rosemary plant, dip the end in rooting compound (available from garden stores), or just place a stem in water until it begins to sprout (changing the water frequently), plant it in soil, and water regularly to prevent the soil from drying out. Alternatively, you can purchase an established plant and put it in a sunny spot with excellent drainage and good air circulation. If you live in a frost-free area, it will survive outside over the winter; otherwise, it is best kept in a planter and brought indoors. Water only when the soil looks and feels dry.

Harvesting Rosemary

To harvest, snip off sprigs as needed once the plant attains a degree of maturity.

Using Rosemary

Remove the rosemary needles from the stem and finely chop to add to your favorite dish, or toss a whole stem directly into a soup, stew, or meat dish; remove before serving. Alternatively, to dry the rosemary, tie one-inch bundles of the herb and hang upside down until dry. Remove the needles from the stems and save them in a spice jar or bag.

Rosemary is a delicious addition to chicken, lamb, or beef, as well as to omelettes and tomato sauces. It can be puréed with olive oil to drizzle over bread in place of butter.

Atherosclerosis Remedy

Preliminary research shows that rosemary has anti-inflammatory effects and holds promise as a natural remedy for atherosclerosis — a chronic inflammation and buildup of plaque in the blood vessels that leads to heart disease, heart attacks, and stroke.[1] According to these scientists, rosemary has the potential to be developed into a natural atherosclerosis medication or functional food.

Brain Booster and Memory Aid

Rosemary's reputation for enhancing memory likely stems from its proven ability to increase blood flow to the brain.[2] Other research proves that rosemary's reputation as a memory aid is well deserved. Researchers at the Department of Pharmaceutical Botany and Plant Biotechnology at Poznan University of Medical Sciences in Poland found that rosemary eaten as part of a regular diet or used as a natural medicine could improve long-term memory in animals. The scientists found that rosemary slowed the degradation of the important neurotransmitter acetylcholine. Among other functions, acetylcholine is involved in the formation of new memories. The scientists suggest that rosemary may be valuable in the prevention and treatment of dementia.[3]

Hair Growth Tonic

Excessive testosterone can cause hair thinning in both men and women. In an article published in the journal *Phytotherapy Research*, scientists found that applying an extract made of rosemary leaves improved hair regrowth in animals affected by excess amounts of testosterone. Scientists found that the rosemary extract appears to block dihydrotestosterone, an active form of testosterone, from binding to androgen receptor sites.[4] See the recipe below for Rosemary Hair Tonic to benefit from rosemary's proven hair-thickening properties.

Prostate Cancer Preventive

In preliminary research, a standardized extract of one of rosemary's active compounds, carnosic acid, demonstrated selective activity against prostate cancer cells, as opposed to healthy cells.[5] While further research is needed to determine rosemary's potential in preventing cancer, this study suggests that it holds promise.

RECIPES

Rosemary Tea

Add two teaspoons of dried rosemary needles or a 4-inch sprig of fresh rosemary to boiled water, and let it sit for 10 minutes. Strain and drink.

Rosemary Hair Tonic

This is a great natural hair rinse for all hair types. If you are interested in promoting hair growth, apply the tonic to your scalp daily for at least a couple of months. Simply pour it over your scalp and leave it in your hair as it dries, or spritz the tonic on your freshly washed, towel-dried hair daily, ensuring that you spritz the scalp.

Makes approximately 1 quart.

1 quart water
Two or three 6-inch sprigs fresh rosemary

In a medium pot, bring the water to a boil. Turn off the heat, add the rosemary sprigs, and cover. Allow to sit for at least 20 minutes. Allow the liquid to cool, then remove the rosemary sprigs and pour the liquid into a bottle. Store the hair tonic in the fridge for up to a week.

Rosemary–Portobello Mushroom Gravy

This gravy is my all-time favorite and worth the minimal effort. Even if you're not a big fan of gravy, I bet you'll love this healthy take on a typically unhealthy food. The rosemary imparts a rich and delicious flavor. What's more, it contains no MSG, artificial colors, or other chemicals that you usually find in gravy made with a packaged gravy mix. Spoon the gravy over your favorite vegetables, grains, chicken, or a baked sweet potato.

Makes 3 to 3½ cups.

3 tablespoons extra-virgin olive oil
½ large onion, sliced
1 sprig rosemary
1 sprig thyme
2 tablespoons gluten-free flour (such as Bob's Red Mill gluten-free flour)
3 cups chicken or vegetable stock, divided
1 teaspoon unrefined salt
1 portobello mushroom, chopped

In a frying pan or medium saucepan, heat the olive oil over low to medium heat until hot but not smoking. Add the onion, rosemary, and thyme, and cook until the onion starts to brown, about 20 minutes. Remove the onion, rosemary, and thyme, and set aside in a bowl. Return the pan to low heat, and whisk in the flour until the mixture forms a thick paste. Allow to brown for 30 to 60 seconds. Then add one cup of the chicken or vegetable stock, whisking constantly until smooth. Whisk in the remaining stock and the salt. Add the onion, rosemary, and thyme back into the gravy, along with the mushroom, and allow to simmer for 10 to 15 minutes. Strain out the onion, mushroom, and herbs. Serve immediately.

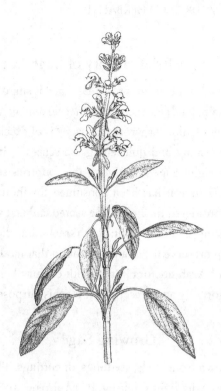

28. Sage

Salvia officinalis

When most people in North America think of sage, they reminisce about Thanksgiving dinners with turkey, stuffing, and all the fixings. But sage deserves much more than once-a-year attention. And when it comes to your brain health, you'll want to give sage a second thought, as it is proving itself to be one of the best natural medicines available for the prevention and treatment of brain diseases.

A Brief History of Sage

In 1597, herbalist John Gerard wrote that sage "is singular[ly] good for the head and brain, [and] quickeneth the nerves and memory."[1] In 1652, herbalist Nicholas Culpeper wrote that sage "is of excellent use to help the memory, warming and quickening the senses."[2] It appears these herbalists were right. Sage is native to the countries surrounding the Mediterranean, where it has been consumed for thousands of years. The Romans considered the herb to be sacred and had special ceremonies for harvesting it. Both the ancient Greeks and the Romans used the herb to help preserve meat, an application that modern science has since validated.[3] Arab doctors in the tenth century believed that sage promoted immortality and prescribed it for this purpose.[4]

Growing Sage

Sage can be grown from seeds, seedlings, or cuttings. The plant prefers a rich, loamy soil with light watering. It can also be grown in pots. Sage plants typically grow to two to three feet tall and need space to grow, so plant them two to three feet apart in garden areas. Plant outdoors after the last frost. Sage likes full sun. In my semiarid desert climate, one species of sage grows wild just about everywhere, even though the conditions tend to be harsh, regularly exceeding 100°F in the summer, with infrequent rain. Most varieties of sage need regular, moderate watering, however. The most commonly available variety for culinary and herbal use is *Salvia officinalis*. The leaves are greyish-green and have a velvety texture.

Harvesting Sage

The leaves are best when harvested before the plant blooms but can be harvested at any time. Hang sprigs upside down to dry, use the herb fresh in your favorite foods, or make an herbal tincture from the fresh leaves.

Using Sage

More than just seasoning for stuffing a turkey, fresh or dried sage is an excellent addition to soups, stews, and chicken dishes. Add it toward the end of the cooking time, as excessive cooking can damage some of its therapeutic compounds. You can also use sage for tea: use one teaspoon of dried herb per cup of hot water, and allow the tea to steep for ten to fifteen minutes before drinking two to three times daily. As with all herbs, fresh sage is best, but feel free to use dried if that's all you have access to. Remember that sage is potent medicine, so if you are on any medication, consult with your doctor before taking it to avoid drug-herb interactions.

While sage is most commonly available as a dried herb, most of the health benefits demonstrated in studies have been achieved using sage oil capsules from the *Salvia lavandulifolia* plant. Because oil constituents vary by brand, follow label directions.

Memory Booster

Sage is a great all-natural memory booster. A British research team conducted a study of sage's therapeutic properties on a group of forty-four adults between the ages of eighteen and thirty-seven. Some participants were given capsules of sage oil, while others were given a placebo of sunflower oil. Results showed that those who took the sage oil performed significantly better on memory tests than those who took the placebo. The people who were given sage as part of the study had improvements in both immediate and delayed word recall scores, as well as mood improvements. Additional research by the same scientific team led them to conclude that sage may also be helpful for those suffering from Alzheimer's disease (see next page).[5]

Healthy Brain Maintenance

While sage is showing promise in the treatment of brain disease, it is also beneficial to the brains of healthy individuals. In research studies, a number of significant effects on cognition were noted with the sage species *Salvia lavandulifolia*. The effects included improvements in both immediate and delayed word recall scores, mood, and overall cognition. It appears to work by inhibiting the enzyme acetylcholinesterase.[6] This enzyme breaks down the essential neurotransmitter acetylcholine, which plays a role in mood regulation, brain-muscle coordination, and the formation of new memories.

Gene Genie

Sage has a proven history of boosting memory and alleviating menopausal and PMS symptoms, but perhaps the most exciting benefit of sage essential oil is that it may actually protect genes from damage. According to a study published in the *Journal of Agricultural and Food Chemistry*, compounds in sage may protect DNA from damage and even stimulate DNA repair in already-damaged cells. While the research is new and the effect has not been tested in humans, this exciting advance could help in the prevention and treatment of genetic diseases as well as diseases with a genetic component, like cancer and heart disease.[7]

Alzheimer's Treatment

Sage's role in limiting the breakdown of the neurotransmitter acetylcholine suggests that the herb may be helpful in the treatment of Alzheimer's disease, since acetylcholine tends to be depleted in Alzheimer's patients.[8] In fact, sage has been found to be so powerful in its ability to treat Alzheimer's disease that the German Ministry of Health is currently considering adding sage as a treatment for Alzheimer's disease to its Commission E Monographs — a compilation of the safety and effectiveness of herbs. While there are various species of sage, the one most commonly found to be beneficial for Alzheimer's disease is *Salvia lavandulifolia*.

Hormone Helper

Because of its estrogen-like properties, sage can help balance hormones in menstruating, nursing, and menopausal women. It may decrease excessive menstruation and lactation and alleviate menopausal symptoms like hot flashes. Inhalation of or massage with diluted sage essential oil is the most direct route of affecting hormones; however, using the herbal extract in tea or tincture form is also helpful.

Multifaceted Healer

The German government already recognizes sage as a treatment for dyspepsia, excessive perspiration, and inflammation of the mouth and nose. (Dyspepsia is a medical term for gas, bloating, burning, and general discomfort of the upper abdomen.)

RECIPE

Brain-Boosting Tea

Take advantage of sage's brain-boosting abilities by enjoying it in tea form. You can add a touch of honey or the natural sweetener stevia if you prefer a sweeter tea. If you're still not wild about the taste of this herbal tea, you can also add one teaspoon of dried peppermint while brewing.

1 cup water
1 teaspoon dried sage leaves or 1 tablespoon fresh sage leaves

In a small saucepan, boil the water. Stir in the sage leaves, cover, and let the mixture steep for at least 10 minutes. Drink one to three cups daily for best results.

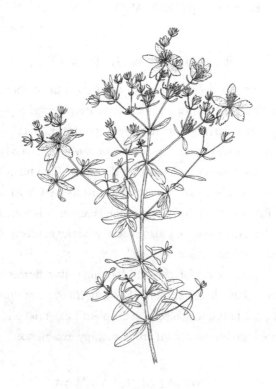

29. St. John's Wort

Hypericum perforatum

St. John's wort often gets a bad rap even in the face of whole volumes of research confirming its effectiveness. It has been shown in many studies to be effective for mild to moderate depression (making it a great herb to keep handy for the winter blues), hormonally linked mood imbalances, and periods of sadness. But St. John's wort has been proven to help many other conditions as well.

A Brief History of St. John's Wort

St. John's wort has been referred to as magical throughout the ages. Its supernatural and spiritual associations are reflected in its scientific name. *Hypericum* derives from the Greek words for "over" (*hyper*) and "apparition" (*eikon*) because the plant was considered so powerful that one whiff caused ghosts and spirits to disappear. The plant's common name, of course, also reveals its connections to the Christian spiritual tradition. Because St. John's Day is the summer solstice, the longest day of the year, the name may also reflect its sunny nature and its ability to lift depressed and anxious moods.[1]

The plant has beautiful, cheerful-looking yellow flowers and leaves that appear to have holes in them. The tiny translucent dots are actually glands, not holes, which release the plant's essential oils and resins when pressed, giving an instant aromatherapy experience.

Growing St. John's Wort

St. John's wort is a perennial plant that grows between one and three feet tall. It grows in most places with moderate sun, but it especially likes sandy soil. Seedlings can be started indoors and transplanted outside after the first frost, when the plants are at least two inches tall. The plant can also be grown indoors if you have enough sunlight and a pot and space that can accommodate fairly tall plants. It usually flowers from late July through August in the second year after planting.

Harvesting St. John's Wort

Use the brilliant yellow flowers of St. John's wort to make tea, tinctures, glycerites, dried flowers, and oil infusions.

Using St. John's Wort

Oil infusions made with St. John's wort can be applied to the skin to treat wounds and to alleviate the pain of diabetic neuropathy. Simply apply the oil two to three times daily until symptoms improve. St. John's wort is also available commercially in dried, capsule, glycerite, or tablet form. For these preparations, follow package instructions, which may vary widely. While some people prefer supplements containing only one of the active ingredients in St. John's wort — hypericin — I prefer tinctures of the plant, since they contain a wider range of active ingredients. Depending on the application, you may need to wait several weeks before noticing results.

Some drugs, including anxiety and depression drugs, antihistamines, digoxin, immune system suppressants, anticonvulsants, blood thinners, birth control pills, antifungals, and calcium channel blockers, can interact with St. John's wort. Check with your pharmacist or doctor before using it in conjunction with any of these medications. Avoid taking it while pregnant or nursing.

Because St. John's wort is so effective for depression, many people consider discontinuing their prescription antidepressants, but it is important never to do so without consulting your physician. You may need to gradually decrease your dose with physician supervision.

Additionally, while St. John's wort is generally safe to use, it can cause photosensitivity in some people, so it is best to avoid direct sun exposure while taking this herb. Some other rare side effects include anxiety, headaches, muscle cramps, sweating, weakness, dry mouth, and skin irritation.

Depression Alleviator

Study after study has proved the effectiveness of St. John's wort in treating depression, particularly mild to moderate depression. Some studies, such as one published in the journal *Phytotherapy Research*, demonstrate that it is as effective as antidepressant pharmaceutical drugs.[2] While there are fewer studies examining St. John's wort's effectiveness against severe depression, one study published in the *Cochrane Database of Systematic Reviews* confirms its value for this purpose.[3] Research published in the *Journal of Zhejiang University Medical Sciences* shows that using St. John's wort in combination with the nutrient quercetin further boosts the antidepressant effects of the herb.[4] And since St. John's wort's safety record is far superior to those of most drugs used for depression, this herb warrants serious consideration.

Anxiety Antidote

Research published in *Phytotherapy Research* also showcases St. John's wort's effectiveness as a natural antianxiety medicine.[5] While the herb's antidepressant and antianxiety effects are often attributed exclusively to hypericin, St. John's wort also contains many other active compounds, including naphthodianthrones, xanthones, flavonoids, and phloroglucinols (hyperforin). Because pharmaceutical drugs tend to contain a single substance that is intended to act on one active mechanism in the body, we often try to compartmentalize herbs in the same way, but they repeatedly show greater effectiveness when their compounds are used together rather than in isolation.

Wound Healer Extraordinaire

St. John's wort flowers have traditionally been macerated into oil to make a natural dressing for healing wounds. Research examining this application found it to be highly effective.[6]

Cancer Answer

Exciting research published in the journal *PLoS One* found that hypericin was highly effective against the invasive cancer melanoma, using three different mechanisms to cause cancer cells to die.[7]

Diabetic Neuropathy Tamer

Research published in the Italian medical journal *Fitoterapia* found that St. John's wort and feverfew flower extracts were highly effective in reducing the pain of diabetic neuropathy. The herbal medicine proved comparable to three different drugs used for the condition.[8]

Migraine Magician

St. John's wort has proved itself effective in the treatment of migraines. Research published in the journal *Phytomedicine* found that St. John's wort blocked pain receptors involved in migraines, making it an effective natural treatment for migraine sufferers.[9]

Menopause Balancer

Research published in the journal *Menopause* found that St. John's wort significantly reduced the frequency and severity of hot flashes in menopausal, perimenopausal, and postmenopausal women.[10] (Perimenopause refers to the ten years prior to menopause. Postmenopause begins one year after periods have altogether stopped.)

Alzheimer's and Dementia Therapy

Swiss scientists published a novel study in the medical journal *Brain Pathology* in which they found that St. John's wort has a protective effect against beta-amyloid plaques linked with Alzheimer's disease.[11] This research, while still in its infancy, shows that the herb has huge promise as a possible treatment for both dementia and Alzheimer's disease.

Parkinson's Disease Aid

Research reported in the medical journal *Cell and Molecular Neurobiology* found that St. John's wort holds promise for the treatment of Parkinson's disease.[12] Unlike many of the drugs used in the treatment of this disease, St. John's wort works on the causal factors linked to the disease. Not only does it reduce inflammation and free radical damage, but it also helps protect the nerves and DNA involved in the condition.

Antioxidant Activator

The same study published in *Cellular and Molecular Neurobiology* also found that St. John's wort is a potent antioxidant, meaning that it destroys harmful free radicals before they can damage the cells and tissues of the body. Because free-radical damage is involved in aging and many diseases, these findings suggest that St. John's wort may have other far-reaching applications.[13]

Restless Leg Syndrome Reliever

New research published in the medical journal *Clinics* suggests that you might also want to consider using St. John's wort to help with restless leg syndrome. Officially known as Willis-Ekbom disease, it is a common condition affecting the nervous system and is characterized by nighttime twitching of the legs. It's not a dangerous condition, but it can be uncomfortable and interfere with quality of sleep and life. One symptom associated with the syndrome is low levels of certain liver enzymes. The study found that St. John's wort extract, taken at a dose of 300 mg daily for three months, boosted these enzymes, and researchers believe that this boost may have a calming effect on restless legs.[14]

RECIPE

Mood Magic Tea

Enjoy St. John's wort tea on a daily basis for at least a week, and you'll be amazed at how it gently and naturally lifts your spirits, particularly if you suffer from depression. As it steeps, it turns a brilliant red color that's as lovely as it is medicinal. You can add a touch of honey or the natural sweetener stevia if you prefer a sweeter tea. If you're still not wild about the taste of this herbal tea, you can also add one teaspoon of dried peppermint while brewing.

1 cup water
1 teaspoon dried St. John's wort flowers or 1 tablespoon fresh
    St. John's wort flowers

In a small saucepan, boil the water. Stir in the St. John's wort, cover, and let the tea steep for at least 10 minutes. Strain. Drink one to three cups daily for best results.

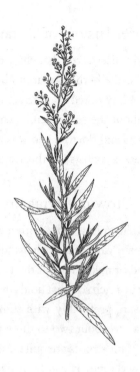

30. Tarragon

Artemisia dracunculus, Artemisia dracunculoides

One of the *fines herbes* of French cuisine, along with parsley, chives, and chervil, tarragon is a frequently overlooked herb in North American cooking. I went most of my life without tasting it, except in the occasional béarnaise sauce, for which tarragon provides the characteristic flavor. Now, however, I always keep a tarragon-infused wine vinegar on hand, as I love the flavor it imparts to homemade salad dressings. Once you learn about the many healing properties of tarragon, you may also wish to keep fresh tarragon in your fridge and some natural remedies made with it in your medicine cabinet.

A Brief History of Tarragon

When the ancient Greeks discovered that chewing tarragon numbs the mouth, they began to use the herb to treat toothaches. In the first century, the Roman writer Pliny noted that tarragon prevented fatigue on long journeys.[1] After about the seventeenth century, tarragon fell out of fashion with herbalists and doctors and was mainly used in French cooking. Even today, few herbalists use this fragrant herb.

Growing Tarragon

Tarragon has a somewhat grassy look, with a slight anise or licorice flavor. There are two main varieties, French and Russian; the leaves of both can be used in food or medicine, but the French variety has a better flavor. It grows best in a rich soil that holds moisture well, and needs moderate amounts of sun, preferably with some shade at the hottest time of the day. It grows to about two to three feet tall both outdoors and in containers. The plant's roots are quite shallow, so be careful not to disrupt them while weeding. It can be grown indoors from seed; seedlings should be planted outdoors after the last frost. Space plants eighteen to twenty-four inches apart, since the plants tend to spread out. Allow the soil to go almost dry between waterings, then soak.

Harvesting Tarragon

It's best to use fresh tarragon leaves or make infusions, tinctures, and vinegars from fresh tarragon, since the herb loses most of its medicinal properties when dried. Fortunately, you can easily preserve the medicinal benefits of the fresh plant in a tincture.

Using Tarragon

In the kitchen, fresh tarragon can be used in vegetable or fish dishes, in white sauces, and with mild cheeses. (Check out my book *The Probiotic Promise* [Da Capo, 2015] to find recipes for suitable mild, dairy-free cheeses.)

Aspirin Alternative

New research in the journal *Pharmaceutical Biology* found that tarragon has significant analgesic effects.[2] The herb also has anti-inflammatory effects, making it an excellent choice in the treatment of pain disorders, including arthritis and fibromyalgia. Additionally, research in the journal *Evidence-Based Complementary and Alternative Medicine* found that sugar increased the levels of many markers for pain and inflammation in animals, but when a tarragon extract was given alongside the sugar, these levels dropped, suggesting analgesic and anti-inflammatory effects comparable to those found in the *Pharmaceutical Biology* study.[3] (While I don't condone the means to obtain the research results, I'd be remiss if I didn't report research findings that may have value to human health.) The latter study used an infusion of tarragon in water.

Blood Pressure Normalizer

According to the well-known botanist James Duke, tarragon contains six different compounds that are linked to lowering high blood pressure.[4]

Toothache Tamer

Because tarragon contains a potent anesthetic compound known as eugenol, it offers all-natural help for toothaches by numbing sensation in the mouth.[5] Use it in moderation for this purpose.

Possible Diabetes Treatment

Exciting preliminary research published in the *Journal of Ethnopharmacology* shows that an extract of tarragon stimulates the release of insulin by the pancreas, which is involved in regulating blood sugar. This new research offers hope for alternative treatments for diabetes sufferers.[6]

RECIPE

Tarragon Apricot Quinoa

This delicious one-pot meal is quick and easy for those times when you're in a rush but want something healthy and delicious to eat. Serves 4.

1 cup quinoa, rinsed
2 cups water
1½ cups kale, finely chopped and packed (or approximately 4 kale leaves, stems removed)
1 carrot, chopped into small chunks
1 small onion, finely chopped
1 tablespoon minced fresh tarragon leaves
1 teaspoon sea salt
3 apricots, fresh or dried, pitted and chopped
1 peach, fresh or dried, pitted and chopped
One 2-inch piece cucumber, chopped
3 tablespoons extra-virgin olive oil
2 tablespoons apple cider vinegar or white wine vinegar

Combine the quinoa, water, kale, carrot, onion, tarragon, and salt in a medium pot. Cover and bring to a boil, then reduce the heat and allow it to simmer on low for 20 to 25 minutes or until the water is absorbed. Remove from the heat. Add the apricot, peach, cucumber, oil, and vinegar, and toss together. Serve immediately.

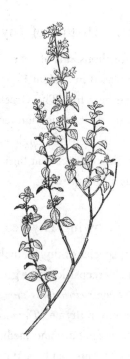

31. Thyme

Thymus vulgaris

Easy to grow indoors or out, thyme is a great addition to your garden and spice cabinet. Not only is it versatile for cooking, but it also has a wide range of therapeutic uses, thanks to the potent antiseptic compound thymol in its leaves.[1] Thyme is an effective and well-known remedy for coughs and sore throats, and now more and more is being discovered about thyme's antimicrobial, anticancer, and other health benefits.

A Brief History of Thyme

Thyme has been in use for thousands of years. It was used in embalming the bodies of the deceased in ancient Egypt, as it was believed to aid their passage into the next life. The Greeks and Romans burned bunches of thyme to purify their homes and temples and to gain courage by inhaling its smoke.[2] In Victorian England, patches of wild thyme were considered irrefutable evidence that fairies had danced the night away where the herb was found growing.[3]

Growing Thyme

There are many different species of thyme, including mother of thyme (*Thymus serpyllum*), which creeps along the ground or stone pathways; golden lemon thyme (*Thymus citriodorus aureus*), which has a strong lemon fragrance; and common thyme (*Thymus vulgaris*), which is the type most often used for its culinary and medicinal purposes. All species of thyme are perennial plants that have tiny leaves and flowers that range from magenta to white. Thyme thrives in full sun in dry, gritty soil. Thyme plants can readily be grown indoors in a sunny window. You'll probably want to grow at least a couple of thyme plants, since they tend to be fairly small. In regions with cold winters, it is best to cover thyme plants with leaves or evergreen boughs in autumn to protect them. Thyme prefers slightly alkaline soil, which you can adjust by adding lime if necessary. Add a slow-release organic fertilizer when planting thyme and again each spring for best results.

Harvesting Thyme

Use sprigs of thyme whole throughout the summer, or cut a sprig and pull the leaves off with your fingers by sliding your thumb and forefinger down the sprig from the top. Once the plants start to flower, you can cut off the top half of the sprigs and hang them upside down in bundles in a dry spot indoors. When the leaves are completely dry, strip them off the stems, and store in a sealed jar. It's best not to cut thyme back by more than half in the fall to avoid killing the plant.

Using Thyme

Thyme leaves or sprigs make a delicious addition to most savory foods, including meat, poultry, and fish dishes. You can also add thyme to soups, stews, and mushroom, vegetable, or bean dishes. Add during cooking to allow the flavor to develop and mellow.

Cough Eliminator

Thyme has been approved by the German government as a treatment for coughs, respiratory infections, bronchitis, and whooping cough.[4] Flavonoids found in the plant have been found to relax muscles in the trachea linked to coughing and inflammation. To make a cough-eliminating tea, add 2 teaspoons of crushed fresh or dried thyme leaves to 1 cup of boiled water. Let the tea steep for 10 to 15 minutes, strain it, and drink.

Fungal Disease Inhibitor

As an increasing number of fungal conditions have become drug resistant, new research about thyme's antifungal activity couldn't have come at a better time. Thyme has shown effectiveness against *Aspergillus* spores — a common type of mold that can cause the lung condition aspergillosis in susceptible individuals.[5] A study in the *Brazilian Journal of Microbiology* found that not only was thyme effective at inhibiting the growth of fungi, but it also increased the potency of the drug fluconazole to kill the disease-causing fungi.[6] However, thyme's own ability to kill fungi may make the drug unnecessary in many cases. Another study in the journal *BMC Complementary and Alternative Medicine* found that thyme is effective against drug-resistant strains of *Candida* fungi — the culprits behind yeast infections.[7]

Back Spasm Soother

According to James Duke, author of *The Green Pharmacy*, thyme's natural essential oils effectively reduced his back spasms.[8] Presumably he applies thyme essential oil in a carrier oil like apricot kernel or sweet almond oil directly to his back or uses it in a bath to penetrate the muscles.

TWELVE WAYS TO USE THYME

Use fresh sprigs or dried leaves of thyme in or with:

Bean dishes (cassoulets)
Beef
Fish
Lamb
Mushroom dishes
Pasta
Pizza
Poultry
Salad dressings
Soups
Stews
Stuffing

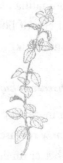

Headache Beater

The medical anthropologist John Heinerman, author of *Heinerman's Encyclopedia of Fruits, Vegetables and Herbs*, recommends drinking thyme tea to treat headaches. He uses one teaspoon of dried thyme per cup of hot water. He also recommends soaking cloths in thyme tea to make a compress to ease aching muscles in the neck, back, and shoulders and to combat tension headaches.[9]

Cancer Fighter

New research in the journal *BMC Research Notes* found that thyme, in combination with Middle Eastern oregano, was effective at inhibiting the proliferation of human leukemia cells, suggesting that the herb may hold potential in the natural treatment of cancer.[10]

RECIPES

Honey-Thyme Cough Syrup

Thyme has been used for many years to help soothe irritated throats and halt coughing. Making your own all-natural thyme cough syrup is quick and easy.

Makes approximately 1½ cups.

1 cup water
2 tablespoons fresh thyme leaves or 2 teaspoons dried thyme leaves
½ cup raw, unpasteurized honey

In a small saucepan, bring the water to a boil. Remove from the heat, add the thyme, and cover. Allow to cool for at least 15 minutes. Strain. Whisk in the honey until mixed. Store in a glass jar in the refrigerator for up to 2 months.

Savory Mushroom and Vegetable Stew

This is a delicious and hearty way to enjoy the flavor and medicinal properties of thyme. While the stew is great on its own, you can also serve it over your favorite biscuits for a real treat. This version is gluten-free and vegetarian, but the flavors work well with chicken or beef, too, if you prefer a meaty stew. The smoked sea salt adds great flavor, but it is also fine to use plain sea salt.

Serves 4.

2 tablespoons extra-virgin olive oil
4 large carrots, cut into ½-inch chunks
2 medium onions, cut into large chunks
6 cloves garlic, peeled
Six 5- or 6-inch sprigs fresh thyme
1 pound white mushrooms, sliced
1 cup peas, fresh or frozen
1 teaspoon smoked sea salt (or regular sea salt)
½ cup water
2 tablespoons gluten-free all-purpose flour

In a medium to large pot or Dutch oven, heat the olive oil over medium heat. Add the carrots and onions, and allow to cook, uncovered, until slightly browned, about 10 minutes. Add the garlic cloves, thyme, mushrooms, peas, and salt. Cover and let the mixture cook until softened, about 10 minutes. In a small bowl, stir the water and flour together until no lumps remain. Stir the water-flour mixture into the pot, and let it cook until it has thickened into a thick gravy. Remove the dish from the heat, and serve immediately.

All-Natural All-Purpose Spray Cleaner

Makes approximately 1 gallon.

1 gallon hot water
½ cup liquid castile soap
10 drops thyme essential oil or ½ cup concentrated thyme
    infusion (3 teaspoons dried thyme to ½ cup boiling water)

Combine all ingredients, and pour into spray bottles. Shake before using.

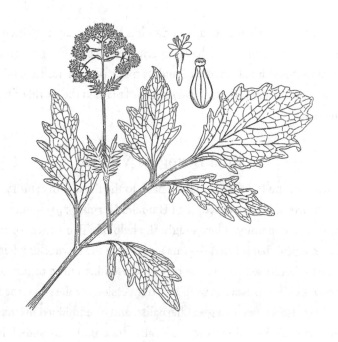

32. Valerian

Valeriana officinalis

Between the ages of nineteen and twenty-two, I managed two health-food stores, one of which I owned. After trying a product called Nerves and Stress, I decided to stock it in the stores. It contained valerian, which is known to relax the nervous system and alleviate the tension linked to stress. Many of my customers who complained of high stress levels reported excellent results with this product.

As more and more exotic herbs from faraway lands have gained popularity in North America, valerian has been largely forgotten, except by a few herbalists who have experienced its benefits. By introducing you to this valuable medicine and its many proven health benefits, I hope to help restore this plant to its rightful place in the world of herbal medicine.

A Brief History of Valerian

The story of the Pied Piper, dating back to the thirteenth century, tells of the efforts of the townspeople of Hameln, Germany, to eliminate rats from their community. They sought the help of a flautist whose music was so magical that it lured the rats away from the town. But when the townspeople refused to pay the piper, he used his music to lure all of the town's children away as well. In older versions of the story, the Pied Piper was also known as a great herbalist, and he combined his musical talents with his herbal ones to magically draw both rats and children out of Hameln. The herb he chose for this endeavor was valerian. Its name comes from the Latin word *valere*, which means "to be strong." The twelfth-century German nun and herbalist Hildegard von Bingen recommended the herb as a tranquilizer and sleeping aid. Native Americans pulverized valerian roots and used them as a treatment for wounds. The herb was included as a tranquilizer in the *U.S. Pharmacopoeia*, an early drug reference book, but by 1942 it had been excluded in favor of synthetic drugs.

Growing Valerian

Valerian grows between three and four feet tall and has clusters of small, beautiful pinkish-purplish and white flowers, making it a lovely addition to a garden space. It can be started from seed indoors about four weeks prior to the first frost or planted directly in the garden. It prefers full sun and moist but free-draining, nutrient-rich soil. Due to its size, it is not really suited for indoor growing.

Harvesting Valerian

Valerian is a perennial herb that may be used after its first year of growth, but it may be preferable to wait until the second year before harvesting the roots in the autumn to obtain enough of the roots for medicinal use.

Using Valerian

Make a tincture from the roots for use as needed, using clean fresh or dried roots prepared according to the directions on page 16. Use one-half to one teaspoon of the tincture at a time to obtain therapeutic benefit, up to two teaspoons daily. While the internet is full of misleading information about adverse interactions of this herb with many drugs, no drug interactions have been reported by the German Commission E, long considered a world authority on the use of herbs. One area of concern has been the possible interaction of valerian with benzodiazepines, a class of drugs used as antianxiety medications (such as Valium), anticonvulsives in epilepsy, and muscle relaxants, which have a long list of potentially harmful side effects. A study published in *BMC Complementary and Alternative Medicine* found that valerian extract had no chemical affinity for benzodiazepine binding sites, suggesting that the herb and the drugs have different mechanisms of activity and that interaction between them is unlikely.[1] Valerian can be used in most of the same ways as benzodiazepines but has numerous other applications and none of the side effects. It can induce sleepiness or drowsiness, but these are typically the intended effects. In extremely rare instances, people have the opposite reaction to valerian, finding that it actually has a stimulating effect. If you discover that you're one of these people, simply discontinue use.

Anxiety Alleviator

The documented antianxiety effects of valerian can be attributed (at least in part) to the compound valerenic acid.[2]

Pain-Relieving Ointment

Some Native Americans made a massage ointment from valerian leaves and sea algae to relieve rheumatic ills, colic, painful menstruation, sprains, and similar conditions.

Fibromyalgia Fix

Fibromyalgia and chronic fatigue syndrome sufferers tend to experience sleep disturbances, such as difficulty falling asleep, interrupted sleep, and a lack of deep sleep. One of the goals in the treatment of fibromyalgia and chronic fatigue syndrome is to improve sleep quality to enable sufferers of these debilitating conditions to sleep more deeply. Deeper sleep allows the body a greater opportunity to heal at the cellular and tissue level. Herbal teas made of valerian tea drunk in the evening can improve sleep quality (provided not so much is drunk as to necessitate nocturnal bathroom visits).

Insomnia Solution

Fibromyalgia and chronic fatigue syndrome sufferers are not the only ones who can benefit from using valerian root tea to help with sleep. You can also use a valerian root tincture if you prefer.

Bipolar Disorder Remedy

Because many people who suffer from the high and low moods of bipolar disorder also suffer from anxiety and insomnia, researchers assessed the potential effectiveness of eleven different herbs as possible natural treatments for these individuals. In an article published in the *Australian and New Zealand Journal of Psychiatry*, the scientists found that valerian showed the greatest promise for the treatment of both anxiety and insomnia in people suffering from bipolar disorder.[3]

Muscle Tension and Cramp Alleviator

Because valerian helps alleviate tension, it is often effective in the treatment of muscle and uterine cramps.

Childhood Restlessness and Hyperactivity Remedy

Researchers who assessed a combination of valerian root extract and lemon balm extract to reduce restlessness, hyperactivity, and impulsiveness in elementary school children found that the blend was effective and also significantly improved concentration after seven weeks of treatment.[4] This remedy may offer an alternative to the use of methylphenidate (Ritalin), which has been shown to increase the risk of depression and anxiety in adulthood. Some scientists believe that Ritalin alters the brain's chemical composition so that it has a lasting effect on mental health. Because the child's brain is growing and developing, the result could be irreversible brain damage.[5] Newer research has also found either short- or long-term use of methylphenidate caused oxidative damage, reduced important brain-protecting enzymes like superoxide dismutase (SOD), and resulted in a significant change in energy metabolism in the brain.[6]

RECIPE

Stress-Soothing Tea

Enjoy valerian's ability to help you relax and cope with stress with this decoction. It's easiest to brew enough for a few days and then heat a cup at a time as desired. You can add a touch of honey or the natural sweetener stevia if you prefer a sweeter tea. As with many of the tea recipes, if you're still not wild about the taste of this herbal tea, you can also add one teaspoon of dried peppermint while brewing.

2 quarts water
3 tablespoons dried valerian root

Combine the water and valerian in a medium to large pot, and bring to a boil. Once it boils, cover the pot, reduce the heat to low, and let the liquid simmer for 45 minutes to an hour. Strain. For best results, drink one to three cups daily, storing any remaining tea in the refrigerator for up to 3 days.

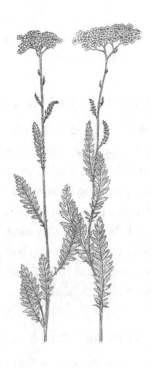

33. Yarrow

Achillea millefolium

Over the years, I've spent many hours harvesting wild herbs from my property, in the forest, or in other natural settings. Yarrow, a lovely herb with feathery leaves and tiny white flowers, is among my favorites. I collect yarrow during the summer to dry and store for use throughout the year or to make into a tincture. One of the reasons I love yarrow is that it is highly effective for many applications. It's also easy to identify and tends to grow somewhat rampant — an indicator of plant strength. After all, plants produce compounds to ensure their survival, and these same compounds are frequently found to be potent medicines that ensure our survival as well.

A Brief History of Yarrow

According to legend, Achilles stopped the bleeding of soldiers' wounds during the Trojan War by applying yarrow leaves (hence the Latin name). He was clearly on the right track, since modern research has confirmed what herbalists have long known: that yarrow has the ability to stop bleeding and reduce pain and inflammation when applied to wounds. It was once called "bad man's plaything," perhaps because it was used to heal cuts and bruises by men who had a habit of brawling.[1] Colonists brought yarrow with them from Europe to North America, where it has since become well established.

Growing Yarrow

Yarrow is fairly easy to grow and can be added to ornamental gardens to fill in spaces, since its clusters of delicate white flowers look a bit like the gypsophila (baby's breath) that is often used in flower arrangements. It is sold as a flowering perennial in many garden stores. Yarrow can be started from seed indoors about six to eight weeks before the last frost, after which it can be planted outside. Give the seedlings about twelve to twenty-four inches of space, since they will spread out. After yarrow has become established, it needs little water or care and is quite drought tolerant, which is one of the reasons it seems to thrive in my semiarid area. However, it is a hardy plant that also thrives in cold-weather climates with more moisture.

Harvesting Yarrow

Cut the mature flowering plants at the base (rather than pulling them out by the roots) and tie the stems in one-inch bundles. Hang them upside down to dry, then store the leaves, stems, and flowers in an airtight container. Alternatively, chop the leaves, stems, and flowers finely to make a yarrow tincture.

Using Yarrow

Menstrual Soother

Yarrow has been approved by the German Commission E as a remedy for the pain of menstrual cramps. Its effectiveness is probably due to several antispasmodic constituents.[2] Some herbal experts, like James Duke, author of *The Green Pharmacy*, also recommend yarrow to help restore periods in women who are not experiencing them (amenorrhea).[3] Of course, if your periods have stopped, you should consult a physician to rule out any serious health conditions.

Urinary Tract Cleanser

The leaves, stems, and flowers of this plant make an effective remedy for cleansing the kidneys. This helps regulate high blood pressure, which is managed largely by the kidneys.

Liver Lover

Yarrow is also a good liver cleanser. Two animal studies have demonstrated its ability to protect the liver from toxic chemical damage. A study published in the journal *Phytotherapy Research* demonstrated its abilities to protect the liver from damage.[4] Use one teaspoon of the dried herb (any combination of leaves, flowers, and stems) per cup of boiling water. Drink one cup three times per day.

Fever Fix

In the herbal world, yarrow is known as a diaphoretic herb — one that induces sweating. The skin is your body's largest detoxification organ, and in some cases of high fever or serious infection, sweating is one of the best ways for the body to reduce its internal temperature and eliminate toxic buildup linked to the infection. Stephen Harrod Buhner, an herbalist and the author of the book *Herbal Antibiotics*, recommends the use of yarrow in combination with potent antibacterial herbs like ginger and echinacea to combat infection. Yarrow's antifever effects are best harnessed by drinking a few cups of yarrow tea daily when you have a fever. Use one teaspoon of the dried herb per cup of boiling water. Drink one cup three times per day.

Chemotherapy Aid

New research in the *European Journal of Oncology Nursing* found that yarrow was highly effective when used as a mouthwash to alleviate irritation and sores in the mucous membranes of the mouth (oral mucositis), which can be symptoms of oral cancers and a serious side effect of cancer chemotherapy.[5]

Antiwrinkle Skin Refresher

According to the *International Journal of Cosmetic Science*, an extract of yarrow applied to the skin significantly reduced the visibility of wrinkles and pores, compared with a placebo and glycolic acid products. Glycolic acid is a substance frequently added to antiwrinkle creams to help remove dead skin cells and give skin a fresher look. Don't be surprised if you start seeing yarrow extracts used in the cosmetics industry in the future.[6]

RECIPES

Yarrow Facial Toner

This easy-to-make facial toner cleanses the skin, tightens pores, and alleviates oily patches, while also helping minimize wrinkles.

    1 cup water
    2 teaspoons dried yarrow
    1 tablespoon witch hazel, available in most health-food stores

In a small saucepan, boil the water. Add the yarrow, and let steep for at least 10 minutes. Let the liquid cool. Strain, add the witch hazel, and pour the mixture into a bottle. Use it in a spray bottle to spritz on skin, or pour a small amount onto a cotton ball and apply to skin. The toner will last for up to one month in the refrigerator.

Yarrow Antiwrinkle Skin Refresher Cream

Yarrow extract is poised to become one of the best antiwrinkle ingredients in the cosmetics industry. But why use wrinkle creams that are full of toxic chemicals and cost a fortune when you can make your own that is much better for your skin and overall health?

As some people experience some skin irritation from yarrow, it is a good idea to test this cream on an inconspicuous area, like the inside of your wrist, and wait at least 48 hours before using elsewhere.

Makes approximately 1¾ cups.

1 cup water
2 teaspoons dried yarrow flowers and leaves or 4 teaspoons fresh
    yarrow flowers and leaves
¾ cup sweet almond oil or apricot kernel oil
2 tablespoons shaved beeswax

Boil the water, and pour it over the yarrow. Cover the mixture, and let it brew for 10 to 20 minutes. Strain out the yarrow, reserving the yarrow-infused water. Set aside.

Pour the oil into a Pyrex measuring cup, and add the shaved beeswax. Set the measuring cup in a saucepan of water that reaches about halfway up the side of the measuring cup. Heat the mixture until the beeswax dissolves, and then remove the measuring cup from the heat immediately. Allow it to cool for a minute or two, but not longer, as the beeswax will begin to harden.

Pour the yarrow-infused water into a blender, cover, and begin blending it on high speed. With the blender running, slowly pour the beeswax mixture through the hole in the blender lid. The mixture will begin to thicken after about three-quarters of the beeswax has been incorporated.

Once all the beeswax has been blended, immediately pour the lotion into a 16-ounce glass jar or two 8-ounce glass jars. Use a spatula to remove any remaining cream from the blender.

The cream lasts about 3 months and is best kept in the refrigerator.

Appendix

A Word to the Wise about Mainstream Herbal Reporting

You may be wondering why media coverage of research on herbal medicines sometimes reports negative, confusing, or contradictory results. Constructing a solid study depends on many factors. The quality and effectiveness of herbal products can vary enormously depending on the herb part used, its preparation, the means of delivery for treating a particular condition (such as internal use or topical application), and the dosage used. Sometimes only a single active ingredient is isolated from an herb and used in a study, when the herb's effectiveness depends on synergistic interactions of compounds found together in the whole plant. Not all studies are constructed by people with sufficient understanding of herbs to obtain positive results.

In some cases, obscure or negative study results may actually be the desired outcome of corporate-sponsored research. The pharmaceutical industry is a multibillion-dollar industry with a substantial interest in safeguarding its profits. Some studies are funded by drug manufacturers who aim to prove that an herb is useless so that people will continue to rely on pharmaceutical options. Such studies typically use a dose that is simply too small to be effective or have too short a duration to yield any significant results.

Notes

Links to the U.S. National Institutes of Health's PubMed database below provide abstracts for the articles and, if available, open-access links to the full text.

Chapter 2: Using Herbs

1 "Make Your Own Herbal Medicines," *Mother Earth News Food and Garden Series, Guide to Healing Herbs*, 16.
2 E. Parker, "The Role of Chief," www.pbs.org/warrior/content/timeline /opendoor/roleOfChief.html.

Chapter 3: Basil (*Ocimum basilicum*)

1 M. Sienkiewicz, M. Łysakowska, M. Pastuszka, W. Bienias, and E. Kowalczyk, "The Potential of Use Basil and Rosemary Essential Oils as Effective Antibacterial Agents," *Molecules* 18 (2013): 9334–51, www.ncbi.nlm.nih.gov /pubmed/23921795.
2 A. Gemechu, M. Giday, A. Worku, and G. Ameni, "In Vitro Antimycobacterial Activity of Selected Medicinal Plants against Mycobacterium tuberculosis and Mycobacterium bovis Strains," *BMC Complementary and Alternative Medicine* 13 (October 2013): 291, www.ncbi.nlm.nih.gov /pubmed/24168665.

3   J. A. Duke, *The Green Pharmacy: The Ultimate Compendium of Natural Remedies from the World's Foremost Authority on Healing Herbs* (New York: St. Martin's, 1997), 312.

4   J. Lv, Q. Shao, H. Wang, H. Shi, T. Wang, W. Gao, B. Song, G. Zheng, B. Kong, and X. Qu, "Effects and Mechanisms of Curcumin and Basil Poly-saccharide on the Invasion of SKOV3 Cells and Dendritic Cells," *Molecular Medicine Reports* 8, no. 5 (2013): 1580–86, www.ncbi.nlm.nih.gov/pubmed/24065177.

Chapter 4: Calendula (*Calendula officinalis*)

1   Cloverleaf Farms, "Calendula," *Herbal Encyclopedia*, www.cloverleaffarmherbs.com/calendula, accessed July 13, 2015.

2   C. E. Stubbe and M. Valerno, "Complementary Strategies for the Management of Radiation Therapy Side-Effects," *Journal of the Advanced Practitioner in Oncology* 4, no. 4 (July–August 2013): 219–31, www.ncbi.nlm.nih.gov/pmc/articles/PMC4093430.

3   M. S. Khairnar, B. Pawar, P. P. Marawar, and A. Mani, "Evaluation of *Calendula officinalis* as an Anti-plaque and Anti-gingivitis Agent," *Journal of the Indian Society of Periodontology* 17, no. 6 (2013): 741–47, www.ncbi.nlm.nih.gov/pubmed/24554883.

4   A. M. Alnuqaydan, C. E. Lenehan, R. R. Hughes, and B. J. Sanderson, "Extracts from *Calendula officinalis* Offer In Vitro Protection against H_2O_2 Induced Oxidative Stress Cell Killing on Human Skin Cells," *Phytotherapy Research* 29, no. 1 (2015): 120–24, www.ncbi.nlm.nih.gov/pubmed/25266574.

5   J. A. Duke, *The Green Pharmacy: The Ultimate Compendium of Natural Remedies from the World's Foremost Authority on Healing Herbs* (New York: St. Martin's, 1997), 185.

6   M. Dinda, U. Dasgupta, N. Singh, D. Bhattacharyya, and P. Karmakar, "PI3K-Mediated Proliferation of Fibroblasts by *Calendula officinalis* Tincture: Implication in Wound Healing," *Phytotherapy Research* 29, no. 4 (2015): 607–16, www.ncbi.nlm.nih.gov/pubmed/25641010.

Chapter 5: Chamomile
(*Chamaemelum nobile*, *Matricaria chamomilla*, *Matricaria recutita*)

1   WebMD, "Topic Overview: What is Chamomile?" www.webmd.com/sleep-disorders/guide/chamomile-topic-overview, accessed September 30, 2015.

2   H. Rahman and A. Chandra, "Microbiologic Evaluation of Matricaria and Chlorhexadine against *E. faecalis* and *C. albicans*," *Indian Journal of Dentistry* 6, no. 2 (2015): 60–64, www.ncbi.nlm.nih.gov/pubmed/26097333.

3   S. A. Seyyedi, M. Sanatkhani, A. Pakfetrat, and P. Olyaee, "The Thera-
peutic Effects of Chamomilla Tincture Mouthwash on Oral Aphthae: A
Randomized Clinical Trial," *Journal of Clinical and Experimental Dentistry*
6, no. 5 (2014): e535–e538, www.ncbi.nlm.nih.gov/pubmed/25674322.
4   H. Sebai, M. A. Jabri, A. Souli, K. Hosni, K. Rtibi, O. Tebourbi, J. El-
Benna, and M. Sakly, "Chemical Composition, Antioxidant Properties, and
Hepatoprotective Effects of Chamomile (*Matricaria recutita* L.) Decoction
Extract against Alcohol-Induced Stress in Rat," *General Physiology and Bio-
physics* 34, no. 3 (2015): 263–75, www.ncbi.nlm.nih.gov/pubmed/25816359.
5   S. Agatonovic-Kustrin, D. Babazadeh Ortakand, D. W. Morton, and
A. P. Yusof, "Rapid Evaluation and Comparison of Natural Products and
Antioxidant Activity in Calendula, Feverfew, and German Chamomile
Extracts," *Journal of Chromatography A* 1385 (2015): 103–10, www.ncbi.nlm
.nih.gov/pubmed/25666499.
6   J. Zhao, S. I. Khan, M. Wang, Y. Vasquez, M. H. Yang, B. Avula, Y.-H.
Wang, C. Avonto, T. J. Smillie, and I. A. Khan, "Octulosonic Acid Deriva-
tives from Roman Chamomile (*Chamaemelum nobile*) with Activities against
Inflammation and Metabolic Disorder," *Journal of Natural Products* 77, no. 3
(2014): 509–15, www.ncbi.nlm.nih.gov/pubmed/24471493.
7   R. Guimaraes, L. Barros, M. Dueñas, R. C. Calhelha, A. M. Carvalho, C.
Santos-Buelga, M. João, R. P. Queiroz, and I. C. F. R. Ferreira, "Nutrients,
Phytochemicals, and Bioactivity of Roman Chamomile: A Comparison
between the Herb and Its Preparations," *Food Chemistry* 136, no. 2 (2013):
718–25, www.ncbi.nlm.nih.gov/pubmed/23122119.

Chapter 6: Chives (*Allium schoenoprasum*)

1   Monterey Bay Spice Company, "Profile: Chives," Herbco, www.herbco
.com/t-chives.aspx, accessed August 17, 2015.
2   "Chives: A Growing Guide," *Rodale's Organic Life*, April 8, 2011, www
.rodalesorganiclife.com/garden/chives-growing-guide.
3   "Profile: Chives."
4   "History of Chives," InDepthInfo, www.indepthinfo.com/chives/history
.shtml, accessed July 20, 2015.
5   "Chives: A Growing Guide."
6   "Profile: Chives."
7   "Profile: Chives."
8   D. Mnayer, A.-S. Fabiano-Tixier, E. Petitcolas, T. Hamieh, N. Nehme, C.
Ferrant, X. Fernandez, and F. Chemat, "Chemical Composition, Antibacterial and Antioxidant Activities of Six Essential Oils from the Alliaceae
Family," *Molecules* 19, no. 12 (2014): 20034–53, www.ncbi.nlm.nih.gov
/pubmed/25470273.

9   H. L. Nicastro, S. A. Ross, and J. Milner, "Garlic and Onions: Their
    Cancer-Prevention Properties," *Cancer Prevention Research* 8, no. 3 (2015):
    181–89, www.ncbi.nlm.nih.gov/pubmed/25586902.

10 Z. Kucekova, J. Mlcek, P. Humpolicek, O. Rop, and P. Valasek, "Phenolic
    Compounds from *Allium schoenoprasum, Tragopogon pratensis,* and *Rumex
    acetosa* and Their Anti-proliferative Effects," *Molecules* 16 (2011): 9207–17,
    www.ncbi.nlm.nih.gov/pubmed/22051932.

11 A. E. Parvu, M. Parvu, L. Vlase, P. Miclea, A. C. Mot, and R. Silaghi-
    Dumitrescu, "Anti-inflammatory Effects of *Allium schoenoprasum* L.
    Leaves," *Journal of Physiology and Pharmacology* (April 2014), www.ncbi
    .nlm.nih.gov/pubmed/24781739.

Chapter 7: Cilantro (*Coriandrum sativum*)

1   A. Aissaoui, S. Zizi, Z. H. Israili, and B. Lyoussi, "Hypoglycemic and
    Hypolipidemic Effects of *Coriandrum sativum* L. in *Meriones shawi* Rats,"
    Journal of Ethnopharmacology 137, no. 1 (September 2011): 652–61,
    www.ncbi.nlm.nih.gov/pubmed/21718774.

2   M. Gong, M. Garige, R. Varatharajalu, P. Marmillot, C. Gottipatti, and
    L. C. Leckey, "Quercetin Up-regulates Paraoxonase-1 Gene Expression
    with Concomitant Protection against LDL Oxidation," *Biochemical and
    Biophysical Research Communications* 379, no. 4 (February 2009): 1001–4,
    www.ncbi.nlm.nih.gov/pubmed/20728021.

3   V. Nair, S. Singh, and Y. K. Gupta, "Evaluation of Disease Modifying
    Activity of *Coriandrum sativum* in Experimental Models," *Indian Journal of
    Medical Research* 135 (February 2012): 240–45.

Chapter 8: Dandelion (*Taraxacum officinale*)

1   R. Bentely and H. Trimen, *Medicinal Plants* (London: J. & A. Churchill,
    1880), 3:159.

2   K. Faber, "The Dandelion: *Taraxacum officinale* Weber," *Pharmazie* 13, no.
    7 (1958): 423–35.

3   A. Mahesh, R. Jeyachandran, L. Cindrella, D. Thangadurai, V. P. Veerapur,
    and D. Muralidhara Rao, "Hepatocurative potential of Sesquiterpene
    Lactones of *Taraxacum officinale* on Carbon Tetrachloride Induced Liver
    Toxicity in Mice," *Acta Biologica Hungarica* 61, no. 2 (June 2010): 175–90,
    www.ncbi.nlm.nih.gov/pubmed/20519172.

4   D. Colle, L. P. Arantes, P. Gubert, S. C. Almeida da Luz, M. L. Athayde,
    J. B. Teixeira Rocha, and F. A. Antunes Soares, "Antioxidant Properties
    of *Taraxacum officinale* Leaf Extract Are Involved in the Protective Effect
    against Hepatotoxicity Induced by Acetaminophen in Mice," *Journal of*

Medicinal Food 15, no. 6 (June 2012): 549–56, www.ncbi.nlm.nih.gov
/pubmed/22424457.

5   B.-R. Lee, J.-H. Lee, and H.-J. An, "Effects of *Taraxacum officinale* on
Fatigue and Immunological Parameters in Mice," *Molecules* 17, no. 11
(November 2012): 13253–65, www.ncbi.nlm.nih.gov/pubmed/23135630.

6   S. J. Chatterjee, P. Ovadje, M. Mousa, C. Hamm, and S. Pandey, "The Ef-
ficacy of Dandelion Root Extract in Inducing Apoptosis in Drug-Resistant
Human Melanoma Cells," *Evidence-Based Complementary and Alternative
Medicine* 2011 (2011), www.hindawi.com/journals/ecam/2011/12904/.

7   S. Sigstedt, C. J. Hooten, M. C. Callewaert, A. R. Jenkins, A. E. Romero,
M. J. Pullin, A. Kornienko, T. K. Lowrey, S. V. Slambrouck, and W. F.
Steelant, "Evaluation of Aqueous Extract of *Taraxacum officinale* on
Growth and Invasion of Breast and Prostate Cancer Cells," *International
Journal of Oncology* 32, no. 5 (2008): 1085–90, www.ncbi.nlm.nih.gov
/pubmed/18425335.

8   P. Ovadje, C. Hamm, and S. Pandey, "Efficient Induction of Extrinsic Cell
Death by Dandelion Root Extract in Human Chronic Myelomonocytic
Leukemia (CMML) Cells," *PLoS One* 7, no. 2 (February 2012): e30604,
http://journals.plos.org/plosone/article?id=10.1371/journal.pone
.0030604.

9   J.-Y. Yoon, H.-S. Cho, J.-J. Lee, H.-J. Lee, S. Y. Jun, J.-H. Lee, H.-H.
Song, et al., "Novel TRAIL Sensitizer *Taraxacum officinale* F. H. Wigg en-
hances TRAIL-induced Apoptosis in Huh7 Cells," *Molecular Carcinogenesis*
(February 2015), www.ncbi.nlm.nih.gov/pubmed/25647515.

10 M. Modaresi and N. Resalatpour, "The Effect of *Taraxacum officinale* Hy-
droalcohol Extract on Blood Cells in Mice," *Advances in Hematology* (2012):
653412, www.ncbi.nlm.nih.gov/pubmed/22844289.

11 H. B. Wang, "Cellulase-Assisted Extraction and Antibacterial Activity of
Polysaccharides from the Dandelion *Taraxacum officinale*," *Carbohydrate
Polymers* 103 (March 2014): 140–42, www.ncbi.nlm.nih.gov/pubmed
/24528711.

12 J. A. Duke, *The Green Pharmacy* (Emmaus, PA: Rodale Press,1997), 414.

13 Duke, *Green Pharmacy*, 49.

Chapter 9: Echinacea (*Echinacea purpurea*, *Echinacea angustifolia*)

1   B. K. McMillan, "About Echinacea," University of Pittsburgh at Bradford,
www.pitt.edu/~cjm6/w98echin.html, accessed August 18, 2015.

2   McMillan, "About Echinacea."

3   A. Schapowal, P. Klein, and S. L. Johnson, "Echinacea Reduces the Risk of
Recurrent Respiratory Tract Infections and Complications: A Meta-analysis

of Randomized Controlled Trials," *Advances in Therapy* 32, no. 3 (March 2015): 187–200, www.ncbi.nlm.nih.gov/pubmed/25784510.

4   D. J. Fast, J. A. Balles, J. D. Scholten, T. Mulder, and J. Rana, "*Echinacea purpurea* Root Extract Inhibits TNF Release in Response to Pam3Csk4 in a Phosphatidylinositol-3 Kinase-Dependent Manner," *Cell Immunology* 297, no. 2 (July 2015): 94–99, www.ncbi.nlm.nih.gov/pubmed/26190752.

5   A. Notarnicola, G. Maccagnano, S. Tafuri, A. Fiore, V. Pesce, and B. Moretti, "Comparison of Shock Wave Therapy and Nutraceutical Composed of *Echinacea angustifolia*, Alpha Lipoic Acid, Conjugated Linoleic Acid, and Quercetin (Perinerv) in Patients with Carpal Tunnel Syndrome," *International Journal of Immunopathology and Pharmacology* 28, no. 2 (June 2015): 256–62, www.ncbi.nlm.nih.gov/pubmed/25953494.

6   D. A. Todd, T. V. Gulledge, E. R. Britton, M. Oberhofer, M. Leyte-Lugo, and A. N. Moody, "Ethanolic *Echinacea purpurea* Extracts Contain a Mixture of Cytokine-Suppressive and Cytokine-Inducing Compounds, Including Some That Originate from Endophytic Bacteria," *PLoS One* 10, no. 5 (May 2015): e0124276, www.ncbi.nlm.nih.gov/pubmed/25933416.

7   D. Kotowska, R. B. El-Houri, K. Borkowski, R. K. Petersen, X. C. Fretté, G. Wolber, K. Grevsen, K. B. Christensen, L. P. Christensen, and K. Kristiansen, "Isomeric C-12 Alkamides from the Roots of *Echinacea purpurea* Improve Basal and Insulin-Dependent Glucose Uptake in 3T3-L1 Adipocytes," *Planta Medica* 80, no. 18 (December 2014): 1712–20, www.ncbi.nlm.nih.gov/pubmed/25371981.

Chapter 10: Elecampane (*Inula helenium*)

1   M. Grieve, "Elecampane," *A Modern Herbal*, www.botanical.com/botanical/mgmh/e/elecamo7.html, accessed August 24, 2015.

2   Grieve, "Elecampane."

3   E. Mazzio, R. Badisa, N. Mack, S. Deiab, and K. Soliman, "High Throughput Screening of Natural Products for Anti-mitotic Effects in MDA-MB-231 Human Breast Carcinoma Cells," *Phytotherapy Research* 28, no. 6 (June 2014): 856–67, www.ncbi.nlm.nih.gov/pubmed/24105850.

4   "Elecampane," *Natural Standard*, http://naturalstandard.com/index-abstract.asp?create-abstract=/monographs/herbssupplements/patient-elecampane.asp, accessed April 21, 2011.

5   J. Y. Seo, J. Park, H. J. Kim, I. A. Lee, J.-S. Lim, S. S. Lim, S.-J. Choi, J. H. Y. Park, H. J. Kang, and J.-S. Kim, "Isoalantolactone from *Inula helenium* Caused Nrf2-Mediated Induction of Detoxifying Enzymes," *Journal of Medicinal Food* 12, no. 5 (October 2009): 1038–45, www.ncbi.nlm.nih.gov/pubmed/19857067.

6   Grieve, "Elecampane."

7   C. L. Cantrell, L. Abate, F. R. Fronczek, S. G. Franzblau, L. Quijano, and
    N. H. Fischer, "Antimycobacteria Eudesmanolides from *Inula helenium*
    and *Rudbeckia subtomentosa*," *Planta Medica* 65, no. 4 (May 1999): 351–55,
    www.ncbi.nlm.nih.gov/pubmed/10364842.

Chapter 11: Feverfew (*Tanacetum* spp.)

1   A. Pareek, M. Suthar, G. S. Rathore, and V. Bansal, "Feverfew (*Tanacetum
    Parthenium* L.: A Systematic Review," *Pharmacognosy Review* 5, no. 9
    (January–June 2011): 103–10, www.ncbi.nlm.nih.gov/pmc/articles/PMC
    3210009/.
2   Pareek et al., "Feverfew."
3   B. Wider, M. H. Pittler, and E. Ernst, "Feverfew for Preventing Migraine,"
    Cochrane Database of Systematic Reviews 2015, no. 4 (April 2015), www.ncbi
    .nlm.nih.gov/pubmed/25892430.
4   L. Mannelli, B. Tenci, M. Zanardelli, A. Maidecchi, A. Lugli, L. Mattoli,
    and C. Ghelardini, "Widespread Pain Reliever Profile of a Flower Extract
    of *Tanacetum parthenium*," *Phytomedicine* 22, nos. 7–8 (July 2015): 752–58,
    www.ncbi.nlm.nih.gov/pubmed/26141762.
5   "Feverfew," Complementary and Alternative Medicine Guide, University
    of Maryland Medical Center, http://umm.edu/health/medical/altmed
    /herb/feverfew.

Chapter 12: Garlic (*Allium sativum*)

1   M. Castleman, *The New Healing Herbs* (New York: Bantam Books, 2002), 286.
2   Castleman, *New Healing Herbs*, 287.
3   J. A. Duke, *The Green Pharmacy* (Emmaus, PA: Rodale Press, 1997), 297.
4   G. M. Volk, A. Henk, and C. M. Richards, "Genetic Diversity among U.S.
    Garlic Clones as Detected Using AFLP Methods," *Journal of the Ameri-
    can Society of Horticulture and Science* 29, no. 4 (February 2004): 559–69,
    http://journal.ashspublications.org/content/129/4/559.
5   Volk et al., "Genetic Diversity among U.S. Garlic Clones."
6   S. Baker, ed., *Herbaceous* (Sydney: Murdoch Books, 2003), 197.
7   Volk et al., "Genetic Diversity among U.S. Garlic Clones."
8   J. I. Rodale, *Encyclopedia of Organic Gardening* (Emmaus, PA: Rodale Press,
    1999), 425.
9   Baker, *Herbaceous*, 197.
10 P. Z. Trio, S. You, X. He, J. He, K. Sakao, and D.-X. Hou, "Chemopreven-
    tive Functions and Molecular Mechanisms of Garlic Organosulfur Com-
    pounds," *Food and Function* 5 (March 2014): 833–44, www.ncbi.nlm.nih
    .gov/pubmed/24664286.

11   Duke, *Green Pharmacy*, 165.

12   Duke, *Green Pharmacy*, 166.

13   Castleman, *New Healing Herbs*, 292.

14   Trio et al., "Chemopreventive Functions."

15   M. Tao, L. Gao, J. Pan, and X. Wang, "Study on the Inhibitory Effect of Allicin on Human Gastric Cancer Cell Line SGC-7901 and Its Mechanism," *African Journal of Traditional, Complementary, and Alternative Medicines* 11, no. 1 (2014): 176–79, www.ncbi.nlm.nih.gov/pubmed/24653574.

Chapter 13: Ginger (*Zingiber officinale*)

1   K. Priebe, "Know Your Spice: A Brief History of Ginger," *Mother Earth Living*, March 16, 2011, www.motherearthliving.com/natural-health /know-your-spice-a-brief-history-of-ginger.aspx.

2   M. Arslan and L. Ozdemir, "Oral Intake of Ginger for Chemotherapy-Induced Nausea and Vomiting among Women with Breast Cancer," *Clinical Journal of Oncology Nursing* 19, no. 5 (October 2015): E92–E97, www.ncbi .nlm.nih.gov/pubmed/26414587.

3   S. Ribel-Madson, E. M. Bartels, A. Borgwardt, C. Cornett, B. Danneskiold-Samsøe, and H. Bliddal, "A Synoviocyte Model for Osteoarthritis and Rheumatoid Arthritis: Response to Ibuprofen, Betamethasone, and Ginger Extract; A Cross-Sectional In Vitro Study," *Arthritis* 2012 (2012): 505842, www.ncbi.nlm.nih.gov/pubmed/23365744.

4   K. C. Srivastava and T. Mustafa, "Ginger (*Zingiber officinale*) in Rheumatism and Musculoskeletal Disorders," *Medical Hypotheses* 39 (1992): 342–48, www.medical-hypotheses.com/article/0306-9877(92)90059-L/abstract.

5   C. D. Black, M. P. Herring, D. J. Hurley, and P. J. O'Connor, "Ginger (*Zingiber officinale*) Reduces Muscle Pain Caused by Eccentric Exercise," *Journal of Pain* 11, no. 9 (September 2010): 894–903.

6   N. S. Mashhadi, R. Ghiasvand, G. Askari, M. Hariri, L. Darvishi, and M. R. Mofid, "Anti-oxidative and Anti-inflammatory Effects of Ginger in Health and Physical Activity: Review of Current Evidence," *International Journal of Preventive Medicine* 4, suppl. 1 (2013): S36–S42, www.ncbi.nlm.nih.gov /pmc/articles/PMC3665023.

7   S. H. Buhner, *Herbal Antivirals: Natural Remedies for Emerging and Resistant Viral Infections* (North Adams, MA: Storey Publishing), 2013.

8   J. J. Gagne and M. C. Power, "Anti-inflammatory Drugs Dramatically Reduce Parkinson's Risk," *Archive of Neurology* 60 (2003): 1059–64, www.ncbi.nlm.nih.gov/pmc/articles/PMC2848103.

9   H. Kabuto, M. Nishizawa, M. Tada, C. Higashio, T. Shishibori, and M. Kohno, "Zingerone [4-(4-Hydroxy-3-Methoxyphenyl)-2-Butanone] Prevents 6-Hydroxydopamine-Induced Dopamine Depression in Mouse

Striatum and Increases Superoxide Scavenging Activity in Serum," *Neuro-chemical Research* 30, no. 3 (March 2005): 325–32, www.ncbi.nlm.nih.gov /pubmed/16018576.

10 B. B. Aggarwal with D. Yost, *Healing Spices* (New York: Sterling Publishing, 2011), 138.

11 Mashhadi et al., "Anti-oxidative and Anti-inflammatory Effects of Ginger."

12 Mashhadi et al., "Anti-oxidative and Anti-inflammatory Effects of Ginger."

13 A. Saxena, K. Kaur, S. Hegde, F. M. Kalekhan, M. S. Baliga, and R. Fayad, "Dietary Agents and Phytochemicals in the Prevention and Treatment of Experimental Ulcerative Colitis," *Journal of Traditional and Complementary Medicine* 4, no 4 (2014): 203–17, www.ncbi.nlm.nih.gov/pmc/articles /PMC4220497.

Chapter 14: Horsetail (*Equisetum arvense*)

1 S. Sierralupe, "Horsetail: Pocket Herbal," *The Practical Herbalist*, www .thepracticalherbalist.com/holistic-medicine-library/horsetail-pocket -herbal, accessed August 27, 2015.

2 A. Howe, "The History of Horsetail," *Alive*, December 5, 2005, www.alive .com/health/the-history-of-horsetail.

3 C. Bessa Pereira, P. S. Gomes, J. Costa-Rodrigues, R. Almeida Palmas, L. Vieira, M. P. Ferraz, M. A. Lopes, and M. H. Fernandes, "*Equisetum arvense* Hydromethanolic Extracts in Bone Tissue Regeneration: In Vitro Osteoblastic Modulation and Antibacterial Activity," *Cell Proliferation* 45, no. 4 (August 2012): 386–96, www.ncbi.nlm.nih.gov/pubmed/22672309.

4 J. Costa-Rodrigues, S. C. Carmo, J. C. Silva, and M. H. Fernandes, "Inhibition of Human In Vitro Osteoclastogenesis by *Equisetum arvense*," *Cell Proliferation* 45, no 6 (December 2012): 566–76, www.ncbi.nlm.nih.gov /pubmed/23106302.

5 D. D. Cetojevic-Simin, J. M. Čanadanović-Brunet, G. M. Bogdanović, S. M. Djilas, G. S. Ćetković, V. T. Tumbas, and B. T. Stojiljković, "Antioxidative and Antiproliferative Activities of Different Horsetail (*Equisetum arvense*) Extracts," *Journal of Medicinal Food* 13, no. 2 (April 2010): 452–59, www.ncbi.nlm.nih.gov/pubmed/20170379.

6 I. I. Tepkeeva, E. V. Moiseeva, A. V. Chaadaeva, E. V. Zhavoronkova, Y. V. Kessler, S. G. Semushina, and V. P. Demushkin, "Evaluation of Anti-tumor Activity of Peptide Extracts from Medicinal Plants on the Model of Transplanted Breast Cancer in CBRB-Rb (8.17) 1Iem Mice," *Bulletin of Experimental Biology and Medicine* 145, no. 4 (April 2008): 464–66, www.ncbi.nlm .nih.gov/pubmed/19110595.

7 A. V. Chaadaeva, I. I. Tenkeeva, E. V. Moiseeva, E. V. Svirshchevskaia, and V. P. Demushkin, "Antitumor Effect of the Plant Remedy Peptide Extract PE-PM in a New Mouse T-Lymphoma/Leukemia Model" (abstract),

Biomed Khimiia 55, no. 1 (January–February 2009): 81–88, www.ncbi.nlm
.nih.gov/pubmed/19351037.

8   Y. Ozay, M. Kasim Cayci, S. Guzel-Ozay, A. Cimbiz, E. Gurlek-Olgun,
and M. Sabri Ozyurt, "Effects of *Equisetum arvense* Ointment on Diabetic
Wound Healing in Rats," *Wound* 25, no. 9 (September 2013): 234–41,
www.ncbi.nlm.nih.gov/pubmed/25867238.

Chapter 15: Juniper (*Juniperus communis*)

1   "Juniper Berry," Wikipedia, https://en.wikipedia.org/wiki/Juniper_berry.
2   V. J. Vogel, *American Indian Medicine* (Norman: University of Oklahoma
Press, 1970), 329–30.
3   "About Growing Juniper," Gardener's Network, www.gardenersnet.com
/tree/juniper.htm, accessed September 1, 2015.
4   F. S. Senol, I. E. Orhan, and O. Ustun, "In Vitro Cholinesterase Inhibitory
and Antioxidant Effect of Selected Coniferous Tree Species," *Asian Pacific
Journal of Tropical Medicine* 8, no. 4 (April 2015): 269–75, www.ncbi.nlm
.nih.gov/pubmed/25975497.
5   O. Cioanca, M. Hancianu, M. Mihasan, and L. Hritcu, "Anti-acetylcholin-
esterase and Antioxidant Activities of Inhaled Juniper Oil on Beta (1–42)
Induced Oxidative Stress in the Rat Hippocampus," *Neurochemical Research*
40, no. 5 (May 2015): 952–60, www.ncbi.nlm.nih.gov/pubmed/25743585.

Chapter 16: Lavender (*Lavandula angustifolia*)

1   M. Nikfarjam, N. Parvin, N. Assarzadegan, and S. Asghari, "The Effects
of *Lavandula angustifolia* Mill. Infusion on Depression in Patients Using
Citalopram: A Comparison Study," *Iranian Red Crescent Medical Journal* 15,
no. 8 (2013): 734–39, www.ncbi.nlm.nih.gov/pubmed/24578844.
2   M. N. Mkolo and S. R. Magano, "Repellent Effects of the Essential Oil of
Lavendula angustifolia against adults of *Hyalomma marginatum rufipes*,"
Journal of the South African Veterinary Association 78, no. 3 (September
2007): 149–52, www.ncbi.nlm.nih.gov/pubmed/18237038.
3   T. Matsumoto, H. Asakura, and T. Hayashi, "Does Lavender Aromatherapy Alleviate Premenstrual Emotional Symptoms? A Randomized Crossover Trial," *BioPsychoSocial Medicine* 7 (May 2013): 12, www.ncbi.nlm.nih
.gov/pubmed/23724853.

Chapter 17: Lemon Balm (*Melissa officinalis*)

1   G. Mazzanti, L. Battinelli, C. Pompeo, A. M. Serrilli, R. Rossi, I. Sauzullo,
F. Mengoni, and V. Vullo, "Inhibitory Activity of *Melissa officinalis* L. on

Herpes simplex Virus Type 2 Replication," *Natural Products Research* 22, no. 16 (2008): 1433–40, www.ncbi.nlm.nih.gov/pubmed/19023806.

2 "Lemon Balm," Complementary and Alternative Medicine Guide, University of Maryland Medical Center, http://umm.edu/health/medical /altmed/herb/lemon-balm.

3 S. Geuenich, C. Goffinet, S. Venzke, S. Nolkemper, I. Baumann, P. Plinkert, J. Reichling, and O. T. Keppler, "Aqueous Extracts from Peppermint, Sage, and Lemon Balm Leaves Display Potent Anti-HIV-1 Activity by Increasing the Virion Density," *Retrovirology* 5 (March 2008): 27, www.ncbi.nlm.nih. gov/pubmed/18355409.

4 "Lemon Balm."

Chapter 18: Licorice (*Glycyrrhiza glabra*)

1 D. Winston and S. Maimes, *Adaptogens: Herbs for Strength, Stamina and Stress Relief* (Rochester, VT: Healing Arts Press, 2007), 175.

2 M. Castleman, *The New Healing Herbs: The Ultimate Guide to Nature's Best Medicines* (New York: Bantam Books, 2002), 394.

3 J. J. Kang, M. A. Samad, K. S. Kim, and S. Bae, "Comparative Anti-inflammatory Effects of Anti-arthritic Herbal Medicines and Ibuprofen," *Natural Product Communications* 9, no. 9 (September 2014): 1351–56, www.ncbi.nlm.nih.gov/pubmed/25918809.

4 J. F. Rebhun, K. M. Glynn, and S. R. Missler, "Identification of Glabridin as a Bioactive Compound in Licorice (*Glycyrrhiza glabra* L.) Extract That Activates Human Peroxisome Proliferator-Activated Receptor Gamma (PPARy)," *Fitoterapia* 106 (October 2015): 55–61, www.ncbi.nlm.nih.gov /pubmed/26297329.

5 M. Lee, M. Son, E. Ryu, Y. S. Shin, J. G. Kim, B. W. Kang, H. Cho, and H. Kang, "Quercetin-Induced Apoptosis Prevents EBV Infection," *Oncotarget* 6, no. 14 (May 2015): 12603–24, www.ncbi.nlm.nih.gov/pubmed/26059439.

6 F. Jiang, Y. Li, J. Mu, C. Hu, M. Zhou, X. Wang, L. Si, S. Ning, and Z. Li, "Glabridin Inhibits Cancer Stem Cell–Like Properties of Human Breast Cancer Cells: An Epigenetic Regulation of miR-148a/SMAd2 Signaling," *Molecular Carcinogenesis* (May 2015) (e-pub), www.ncbi.nlm.nih.gov/ pubmed/25980823.

7 J. A. Duke, *The Green Pharmacy* (Emmaus, PA: Rodale Press, 1997), 520.

8 Lee et al., "Quercetin-Induced Apoptosis."

9 D. B. Mowrey, *The Scientific Validation of Herbal Medicine: How to Remedy and Prevent Disease with Herbs, Vitamins, Minerals, and Other Nutrients* (Lincolnwood, IL: Keats Publishing, 1986), 172.

Chapter 19: Milk Thistle (*Silybum marianum*)

1   M. Castleman, *The New Healing Herbs* (New York: Bantam Books, 2002), 416.

2   "Milk Thistle," Agriculture, Government of Saskatchewan, www .agriculture.gov.sk.ca/Default.aspx?DN=9f9ebf1f-6e30-451f-a1ea -d711a59f5d21.

3   "Milk Thistle," Complementary and Alternative Medicine Guide, University of Maryland Medical Center, https://umm.edu/health/medical /altmed/herb/milk-thistle.

4   "Milk Thistle for Professionals (PDQ)," Complementary and Alternative Medicine, National Cancer Institute, www.cancer.gov/about-cancer /treatment/cam/hp/milk-thistle-pdq.

5   X. Williams, *The Herbal Detox Plan* (Carlsbad, CA: Hay House, 2003), 129.

6   J. A. Duke, *Dr. Duke's Essential Herbs* (New York: St. Martin's, 2001), 201–2.

7   Duke, *Dr. Duke's Essential Herbs*, 201–2.

8   F. DiPierro, I. Bellone, G. Rapacioli, and P. Putignano, "Clinical Role of a Fixed Combination of Standardized *Berberis aristata* and *Silybum marianum* Extracts in Diabetic and Hypercholestolemic Patients Intolerant to Statins," *Diabetes, Metabolic Syndrome, and Obesity: Targets and Therapy* 8 (February 2015): 89–96, www.ncbi.nlm.nih.gov/pubmed/25678808.

Chapter 20: Mullein (*Verbascum thapsus*)

1   S. Sepahi, A. Ghorani-Azam, S. Sepahi, A. Asoodeh, and S. Rostami, "In Vitro Study to Evaluate Antibacterial and Non-haemolytic Activities of Four Iranian Medicinal Plants," *West Indian Medical Journal* 63, no. 4 (August 2014): 289–93, www.ncbi.nlm.nih.gov/pubmed/25429470.

2   Z. F. Kashan, M. Arbabi, M. Delavari, H. Hooshyar, M. Taghizadeh, and Z. Joneydy, "Effects of *Verbascum thapsus* Ethanol Extract on Induction of Apoptosis in *Trichomonas vaginalis* In Vitro," *Infectious Disorders Drug Targets* 15, no. 2 (2015): 125–30, www.ncbi.nlm.nih.gov/pubmed/26239850.

3   E. McCarthy and J. M. O'Mahony, "What's in a Name? Can Mullein Weed Beat TB Where Modern Drugs Are Failing?" *Evidence-Based Complementary and Alternative Medicine* 2011 (2011): 239237, www.ncbi.nlm.nih.gov /pmc/articles/PMC2952292.

4   N. Ali, S. W. Ali Shah, I. Shah, G. Ahmed, M. Ghias, I. Khan, and W. Ali, "Antihelmintic and Relaxant Activities of *Verbascum thapsus* Mullein," *BMC Complementary and Alternative Medicine* 12 (March 2012): 29, www.ncbi.nlm .nih.gov/pubmed/22463730.

Chapter 21: Nettles (*Urtica dioica*)

1   B. Roschek Jr., R. C. Fink, M. McMichael, and R. S. Alberte, "Nettle Extract (*Urtica dioica*) Affects Key Receptors and Enzymes Associated with Allergic Rhinitis," *Phytotherapy Research* 23, no. 7 (July 2009): 920–26, www.ncbi.nlm.nih.gov/pubmed/19140159.

2   S. S. Patel and M. Udayabanu, "Effect of *Urtica doica* on Memory Dysfunction and Hypoalgesia in an Experimental Model of Diabetic Neuropathy," *Neuroscience Letters* 552 (September 2013): 114–19, www.ncbi.nlm.nih.gov/pubmed/23916662.

3   "Stinging Nettle," Complementary and Alternative Medicine Guide, University of Maryland Medical Center, http://umm.edu/health/medical/altmed/herb/stinging-nettle.

4   "Stinging Nettle."

5   "Stinging Nettle."

6   Roschek et al., "Nettle Extract."

Chapter 22: Oregano (*Origanum vulgare*)

1   "Oregano," InDepthInfo, www.indepthinfo.com/oregano/history.shtml, accessed October 15, 2015.

2   M. Fournomiti, A. Kimbaris, I. Mantzourani, S. Plessas, I. Theodoridou, I. Papaemmanouil, A. Alexopoulos, et al., "Antimicrobial Activity of Essential Oils of Cultivated Oregano (*Origanum vulgare*), Sage (*Salvia officinalis*), and Thyme (*Thymus vulgaris*) against Clinical Isolates of *Escherichia coli*, *Klebsiella oxytoca*, and *Klebsiella pneumoniae*," *Microbial Ecology in Health and Disease* 26, no. 10 (2015): 3402, www.ncbi.nlm.nih.gov/pubmed/25881620.

3   Shahab Quereshi, "*Klebsiella* Infections," Medscape, http://emedicine.medscape.com/article/219907-overview#a6, accessed October 15, 2015.

4   G. Magi, E. Marini, and B. Facinelli, "Antimicrobial Activity of Essential Oils and Carvacrol, and Synergy of Carvacrol and Erythromycin, against Clinical, Erythromycin-Resistant Group A Streptococci," *Frontiers in Microbiology* 6 (March 2015): 165, www.ncbi.nlm.nih.gov/pubmed/25784902.

5   For example, see M. Vujicic et al., "Methanolic Extract of *Origanum vulgare* Ameliorates Type 1 Diabetes through Antioxidant, Anti-inflammatory and Anti-apoptotic Activity," *British Journal of Nutrition* 113, no. 5 (March 2015): 770–82, www.ncbi.nlm.nih.gov/pubmed/25671817.

6   J. A. Duke, *The Green Pharmacy* (Emmaus, PA: Rodale Press, 1997), 310.

7   K. R. Begnini, F. Nedel, R. G. Lund, P. H. Carvalho, M. R. Rodrigues, F. T. Beira, and F. A. Del-Pino, "Composition and Anti-proliferative Effect of Essential Oil of *Origanum vulgare* against Tumor Line Cells," *Journal of Medicinal Food* 17, no. 10 (October 2014): 1129–33, www.ncbi.nlm.nih.gov/pubmed/25230257.

8   M. Marrelli, B. Cristaldi, F. Menichini, and F. Conforti, "Inhibitory Effects
    of Wild Dietary Plants on Lipid Peroxidation and on the Proliferation of
    Human Cancer Cells," *Food and Chemical Toxicology* 86 (September 2015):
    16–24, www.ncbi.nlm.nih.gov/pubmed/26408343.
9   Duke, *Green Pharmacy*, 82.
10 Duke, *Green Pharmacy*, 225.

Chapter 23: Parsley (*Petroselinum sativum*)

1   T. Ombrello, "Plant of the Week: Parsley," Union County Community
    College, http://faculty.ucc.edu/biology-ombrello/pow/parsley.htm,
    accessed September 10, 2015.
2   Ombrello, "Plant of the Week: Parsley."
3   "Parsley," *The Old Farmer's Almanac*, www.almanac.com/plant/parsley,
    accessed September 10, 2015.
4   E. L. Tang, J. Rajarajeswaran, S. Fung, and M. S. Kanthimathi, "*Petroseli-
    num crispum* Has Antioxidant Properties, Protects against DNA Damage
    and Inhibits Proliferation and Migration of Cancer Cells," *Journal of
    the Science of Food and Agriculture* 95, no. 13 (October 2015): 2763–71,
    www.ncbi.nlm.nih.gov/pubmed/25582089.
5   R. Zamora-Ros, N. G. Forouhi, S. J. Sharp, C. A. González, B. Buijsse, M.
    Guevara, N. J. Wareham, et al., "Dietary Intakes of Individual Flavanols
    and Flavonols Are Inversely Associated with Incident Type 2 Diabetes
    in European Populations," *Journal of Nutrition* 144, no. 3 (2014): 335–343,
    www.ncbi.nlm.nih.gov/pubmed/24368432.
6   Myricetin content of foods, Merschat.com database, http://nutrition
    .merschat.com/foods-by-nutrient.cgi?Nutr_No=788, accessed September
    11, 2015.
7   N. G. Forouhi et al., "Differences in the Prospective Association between
    Individual Plasma Phospholipid Saturated Fatty Acids and Incident Type
    2 Diabetes: The EPIC-InterAct Case-Cohort Study," *Lancet Diabetes and
    Endocrinology* 2, no. 10 (October 2014): 810–18, www.ncbi.nlm.nih.gov
    /pubmed/25107467.
8   J. Saeidi, H. Bozorgi, A. Zendehdel, and J. Mehrzad, "Therapeutic Effects
    of Aqueous Extracts of *Petroselinum sativum* on Ethylene Glycol-Induced
    Kidney Calculi in Rats," *Urology Journal* 9, no. 1 (Winter 2012): 361–66,
    www.ncbi.nlm.nih.gov/pubmed/22395833.

Chapter 24: Peppermint (*Mentha x piperita*)

1   "Peppermint," The World's Healthiest Foods, www.whfoods.com/genpage
    .php?tname=foodspice&dbid=102.

2 "Mint: A Growing Guide," *Rodale's Organic Life*, www.rodalesorganiclife
   .com/garden/mint-growing-guide.

3 "Peppermint."

4 Dominion Herbal College, *Dominion Herbal College: Chartered Herbalist
   Course*, Book 2 (Burnaby, BC: Dominion Herbal College, 1999), pp. L5, 16.

5 J. A. Duke, *The Green Pharmacy* (Emmaus, PA: Rodale Press, 1997), 473.

6 Duke, *Green Pharmacy*, 411.

7 Duke, *Green Pharmacy*, 253–54.

8 J. Heinerman, *Healing Herbs and Spices* (New York: Reward Books, 1996),
   333.

9 "Professor's Study Finds that Peppermint and Cinnamon Lower Frustration and Increase Alertness in Drivers," Wheeling Jesuit University, www
   .wju.edu/about/adm_news_story.asp?iNewsID=1484, accessed December
   10, 2014.

Chapter 25: Plantain (*Plantago major*)

1 "Plantain," Prairieland Herbs, www.prairielandherbs.com/plantain.htm,
   accessed December 10, 2014.

2 C. Staiger, "Comfrey: A Clinical Overview," *Phytotherapy Research* (October 2012), www.ncbi.nlm.nih.gov/pmc/articles/PMC3491633.

3 Y. M. Kim, U.-C. Sim, Y. Shin, and Y. Kim Kwon, "Aucubin Promotes
   Neurite Growth in Neural Stem Cells and Axonal Regeneration in Sciatic
   Nerves," *Experimental Neurobiology* 23, no. 3 (September 2014): 238–45,
   www.ncbi.nlm.nih.gov/pubmed/25258571.

4 M. R. deOliveria, S. F. Nabavi, S. Habtemariam, I. Erdogan Orhan, M.
   Daglia, and S. M. Nabavi, "The Effects of Baicalein and Baicalin on Mito-
   chondrial Function and Dynamics: A Review," *Pharmacology Research* 100
   (October 2015): 296–308, www.ncbi.nlm.nih.gov/pubmed/26318266.

5 J. Liu, "Pharmacology of Oleanic Acid and Ursolic Acid," *Journal of Ethnopharmacology* 49, no. 2 (December 1995): 57–68, www.ncbi.nlm.nih.gov
   /pubmed/8847885.

6 "Plantain."

7 M. Galvez, C. Martín-Cordero, M. López-Lázaro, F. Cortés, and M. J.
   Ayuso, "Cytotoxic Effect of *Plantago* Spp. on Cancer Cell Lines," *Journal of
   Ethnopharmacology* 88, nos. 2–3 (October 2003): 125–30, www.ncbi.nlm.nih
   .gov/pubmed/12963131.

Chapter 26: Red Clover (*Trifolium pratense*)

1 M.Castleman, *The New Healing Herbs: The Ultimate Guide to Nature's Best
   Medicines* (New York: Bantam Books, 2002), 484.

2 R. Zhou, L. Xu, M. Ye, M. Liao, H. Dum, and H. Chen, "Formononetin
    Inhibits Migration and Invasion of MDA-MB-231 and 4T1 Breast Cancer
    Cells by Suppressing MMP-2 and MMP-9 through PI3K/AKT Signaling
    Pathways," *Hormone and Metabolic Research* 46, no. 11 (October 2014):
    753–60, www.ncbi.nlm.nih.gov/pubmed/24977660.
3 Castleman, *New Healing Herbs*, 484.
4 P. B. Clifton-Bligh, M.-L. Nery, R. J. Clifton-Bligh, S. Visvalingam,
    G. R. Fulcher, K. Byth, and R. Baber, "Red Clover Isoflavones Enriched
    with Formononentin Lower Serum LDL Cholesterol: A Randomized,
    Double-Blind, Placebo-Controlled Study," *European Journal of Clinical
    Nutrition* 69, no. 1 (January 2015): 134–42, www.ncbi.nlm.nih.gov
    /pubmed/25369831.
5 I. Kaczmarczyk-Sedlak, W. Wojnar, M. Zych, E. Ozimina-Kamińska, J.
    Taranowicz, and A. Siwek, "Effect of Formononetin on Mechanical Prop-
    erties and Chemical Composition of Bones in Rats with Ovariectomy-
    Induced Osteoporosis," *Evidence-Based Complementary and Alternative
    Medicine: eCAM* (2013): 457052, www.ncbi.nlm.nih.gov/pubmed/23762138.

Chapter 27: Rosemary (*Rosmarinus officinalis*)

1 I. G. Chae, M. Yu, N.-K. Im, Y. T. Jung, J. Lee, K.-S. Chun, and I.-S. Lee,
    "Effect of *Rosmarinus officinalis* L. on MMP-9, MCP-1 Levels, and Cell Mi-
    gration in RAW 267.4 and Smooth Muscle Cells," *Journal of Medicinal Food*
    15, no. 10 (October 2012): 879–86, www.ncbi.nlm.nih.gov/pmc/articles
    /PMC3466913.
2 "Rosemary," The World's Healthiest Foods, www.whfoods.com/genpage
    .php?tname=foodspice&dbid=75, accessed September 22, 2015.
3 M. Ozarowski, P. L. Mikolajczak, A. Bogacz, A. Gryszczynska, M.
    Kujawska, J. Jodynis-Liebert, A. Piasecka, H. Napieczynska, et al.,
    "*Rosmarinus officinalis* L. Leaf Extract Improves Memory Impairment and
    Affects Acetylcholinesterase and Butyrylcholinesterase Activities in Rat
    Brain," *Fitoterapia* 91 (December 2013): 261–71, www.ncbi.nlm.nih.gov
    /pubmed/24080468.
4 K. Murata, K. Noguchi, M. Kondo, M. Onishi, N. Watanabe, K. Okamura,
    and H. Matsuda, "Promotion of Hair Growth by *Rosmarinus officinalis*
    Leaf Extract," *Phytotherapy Research* 27, no. 2 (February 2013): 212–17,
    www.ncbi.nlm.nih.gov/pubmed/22517595.
5 S. M. Petiwala, S. Berhe, G. Li, A. G. Puthenveetil, O. Rahman, L. Nonn,
    and J. J. Johnson, "Rosemary (*Rosmarinus officinalis*) Extract Modulates
    CHOP/GADD153 to Promote Androgen Receptor Degradation and
    Decreases Xenograft Tumor Growth," *PLoS One* 9, no. 3 (March 2014):
    e89772, www.ncbi.nlm.nih.gov/pubmed/24598693.

Chapter 28: Sage (*Salvia officinalis*)

1 J. Gerard, *The Herball or Generall Historie of Plantes* (London: John Norton, 1597), 624.
2 N. Culpeper, *Culpeper's Complete Herbal* (1653; reprint, London: Richard Evans, 1816), 162.
3 "Sage," The World's Healthiest Foods, www.whfoods.com/genpage .php?tname=foodspice&dbid=76, accessed October 1, 2015.
4 "Sage."
5 "Sage May Help Alzheimers Sufferers," *Independent*, August 29, 2003.
6 P. J. Houghton, "Activity and Constituents of Sage Relevant to the Potential Treatment of Symptoms of Alzheimer's Disease," *Herbalgram: The Journal of the American Botanical Council* 61 (2004): 38–53, http://cms.herbalgram.org/herbalgram/issue61/article2643.html.
7 A. A. Ramos, A. Azqueta, C. Pereira-Wilson, and A. R. Collins, "Polyphenolic Compounds from *Salvia* Species Protect Cellular DNA from Oxidation and Stimulate DNA Repair in Cultured Human Cells," *Journal of Agricultural and Food Chemistry* 58, no. 12 (June 2010): 7465–71, www .ncbi.nlm.nih.gov/pubmed/20486687.
8 "Sage May Help Alzheimers Sufferers."

Chapter 29: St. John's Wort (*Hypericum perforatum*)

1 R. Nelson, "St. John's Wort," Dr. Christopher's Herbal Legacy, www.herballegacy.com/Nelson_History.html, accessed July 1, 2015.
2 E. Russo, F. Scicchitano, B. J. Whalley, C. Mazzitello, M. Ciriaco, S. Esposito, M. Patanè, et al., "*Hypericum perforatum*: Pharmacokinetic, Mechanism of Action, Tolerability, and Clinical Drug-Drug Interactions," *Phytotherapy Research* 28, no. 5 (May 2014): 643–55, www.ncbi.nlm.nih .gov/pubmed/23897801.
3 K. Linde, M. M. Berner, and L. Kriston, "St. John's Wort for Major Depression," *Cochrane Database of Systematic Reviews* 4 (October 2008): CD000448, www.ncbi.nlm.nih.gov/pubmed/18843608.
4 J. Liu, Y. Fang, Z. Wei, X. Yang, and L. Zeng, "Synergic Antidepressive Effect of Quercetin and *Hypericum perforatum* Extract in Mice" (abstract), *Zhejiang Da Xue Xue Bao Yi Xue Ban* 42, no. 6 (November 2013): 615–19, www.ncbi.nlm.nih.gov/pubmed/24421225.
5 Russo et al., "*Hypericum perforatum*."
6 A. I. Prisacaru, C. V. Andriţoiu, C. Andriescu, E. C. Hăvârneanu, M. Popa, A. G. Motoc, and A. Sava, "Evaluation of the Wound-Healing Effect of a Novel *Hypericum perforatum* Ointment in Skin Injury," *Romanian Journal of Morphology and Embryology* 54, no. 4 (2013): 1053–59, www.ncbi.nlm.nih .gov/pubmed/24399001.

7   B. Kleemann, B. Loos, T. J. Scriba, D. Lang, and L. M. Davids, "St. John's Wort (*Hypericum perforatum* L.) Photomedicine: Hypericin-Photodynamic Therapy Induces Metastatic Melanoma Cell Death," *PLoS One* 9, no. 7 (July 2014): e103762, www.ncbi.nlm.nih.gov/pubmed/25076130.

8   N. Galeotti, A. Maidecchi, L. Mattoli, M. Burico, and C. Ghelardini, "St. John's Wort Seed and Feverfew Flower Extracts Relieve Painful Diabetic Neuropathy in a Rat Model of Diabetes," *Fitoterapia* 92 (January 2014): 23–33, www.ncbi.nlm.nih.gov/pubmed/24125916.

9   N. Galeotti and C. Ghelardini, "St. John's Wort Reversal of Meningeal Nociception: A Natural Therapeutic Perspective for Migraine Pain," *Phytomedicine* 20, no. 10 (July 2013): 930–38, www.ncbi.nlm.nih.gov /pubmed/23578992.

10 K. Abdali, M. Khajehei, and H. R. Tabatabaee, "Effect of St. John's Wort on Severity, Frequency, and Duration of Hot Flashes in Premenopausal, Perimenopausal, and Post-menopausal Women: A Randomized, Double-Blind, Placebo-Controlled Study," *Menopause* 17, no. 2 (March 2010): 326–31, www.ncbi.nlm.nih.gov/pubmed/20216274.

11 A. Brenn, M. Grube, G. Jedlitschky, A. Fischer, B. Strohmeier, M. Eiden, M. Keller, M. H. Groschup, and S. Vogelgesang, "St. John's Wort Reduces Beta Amyloid Accumulation in a Double Transgenic Alzheimer's Disease Mouse-Model Role of P-Glycoprotein," *Brain Pathology* 24, no. 1 (January 2014): 18–24, www.ncbi.nlm.nih.gov/pubmed/23701205.

12 Z. Kiasalari, T. Baluchnejadmojarad, and M. Roghani, "*Hypericum perforatum* Hydroalcoholic Extract Mitigates Motor Dysfunction and Is Neuroprotective in Intrastriatal 6-Hydroxydopamine Rat Model of Parkinson's Disease," *Cellular and Molecular Neurobiology*, June 29, 2015 (e-pub), www.ncbi.nlm.nih.gov/pubmed/26119304.

13 Kiasalari et al., "*Hypericum perforatum* Hydroalcoholic Extract."

14 J. C. Pereira Jr., M. Pradella-Hallinan, and R. C. Alves, "St. John's Wort, an Herbal Inducer of the Cytochrome P4503A4 Isoform, May Alleviate Symptoms of Willis-Eksbom's Disease," *Clinics (São Paulo)* 68, no. 4 (April 2013): 469–74, www.ncbi.nlm.nih.gov/pmc/articles/PMC3634959.

Chapter 30: Tarragon
(*Artemisia dracunculus, Artemisia dracunculoides*)

1   M. Castleman, *The New Healing Herbs: The Ultimate Guide to Nature's Best Medicines* (New York: Bantam Books, 2002), 552.

2   A. Eidi, S. Oryan, J. Zaringhalam, and M. Rad, "Antinociceptive and Anti-inflammatory Effects of the Aerial Part of *Artemisia dracunculus* in Mice," *Pharmaceutical Biology* (June 2015): 1–6 (e-pub), www.ncbi.nlm.nih .gov/pubmed/26079854.

3   S. Mohammad Reza, M. Hamideh, and S. Zahra, "The Nociceptive and Anti-inflammatory Effects of *Artemisia Dracunculus* L. Aqueous Extract on Fructose-Fed Male Rats," *Evidence-Based Complementary and Alternative Medicine* 2015 (2015): 895417 (e-pub), www.ncbi.nlm.nih.gov/pubmed /26170888.

4   J. A. Duke, *The Green Pharmacy* (Emmaus, PA: Rodale Press, 1997), 312.

5   Castleman, *New Healing Herbs*, 552.

6   S. Aqqarwal, G. Shailendra, D. M. Ribnicky, D. Burk, N. Karki, and M. S. Q. Wang, "An Extract of *Artemisia dracunculus* L. Stimulates Insulin Secretion from Beta Cells, Activates AMPK, and Suppresses Inflammation," *Journal of Ethnopharmacology* 170 (July 2015): 98–105, www.ncbi .nlm.nih.gov/pubmed/25980421.

Chapter 31: Thyme (*Thymus vulgaris*)

1   B. Dunn, "A Brief History of Thyme," History.com, www.history.com /news/hungry-history/a-brief-history-of-thyme, accessed October 2, 2015.

2   Dunn, "Brief History of Thyme."

3   Dunn, "Brief History of Thyme."

4   J. A. Duke, *The Green Pharmacy* (Emmaus, PA: Rodale Press, 1997), 36.

5   "Aspergillosis," Centers for Disease Control and Prevention, October 2, 2015, www.cdc.gov/fungal/diseases/aspergillosis/index.html?s_cid =cs_748.

6   M. S. Khan, I. Ahmad, and S. S. Cameotra, "*Carum copticum* and *Thymus vulgaris* Oils Inhibit Virulence in *Trichophyton rubrum* and *Aspergillus* Spp.," *Brazilian Journal of Microbiology* 45, no. 2 (August 2014): 523–31, www.ncbi .nlm.nih.gov/pubmed/25242937.

7   M. S. Khan, I. Ahmad, S. S. Cameotra, and F. Botha, "Sub MICs of *Carum copticum* and *Thymus vulgaris* Influence Virulence Factors and Biofilm Formation in *Candida* Spp.," *BMC Complementary and Alternative Medicine* 14 (September 2014): 337, www.ncbi.nlm.nih.gov/pubmed/25220750.

8   Duke, *Green Pharmacy*, 36.

9   Duke, *Green Pharmacy*, 289.

10 B. M. Ayesh, A. A. Abed, and D. M. Faris, "In Vitro Inhibition of Human Leukemia THP-1 Cells by *Origanum syriacum* L. and *Thymus vulgaris* L. Extracts," *BMC Research Notes* 7 (September 2014): 612, www.ncbi.nlm.nih .gov/pubmed/25194985.

Chapter 32: Valerian (*Valeriana officinalis*)

1   A. Becker, F. Felgentreff, H. Schröder, B. Meier, and A. Brattström, "The Anxiolytic Effects of a Valerian Extract Is Based on Valerenic Acid," *BMC Complementary and Alternative Medicine* 14 (July 2014): 267, www.ncbi.nlm .nih.gov/pubmed/25066015.

2   Becker et al., "Anxiolytic Effects."

3   J. H. Baek, A. A. Nierenber, and G. Kinrys, "Clinical Applications of Herbal Medicines for Anxiety and Insomnia: Targeting Patients with Bipolar Disorder," *Australian and New Zealand Journal of Psychiatry* 48, no. 8 (August 2014): 705–15, www.ncbi.nlm.nih.gov/pubmed/24947278.

4   J. Gromball, F. Beschorner, C. Wantzen, U. Paulsen, and M. Burkart, "Hyperactivity, Concentration Difficulties, and Impulsiveness Improve during Seven Weeks' Treatment with Valerian Root and Lemon Balm Extracts in Primary School Children," *Phytomedicine* 21, nos. 8–9 (July–August, 2014): 1098–103, www.ncbi.nlm.nih.gov/pubmed/24837472.

5   Pravin Char, "Ritalin 'May Cause Damage to Brains,'" *ThisisLondon*, December 17, 2003.

6   C. M. Comim, K. M. Gomes, G. Z. Réus, F. Petronilho, G. K. Ferreira, E. L. Streck, F. Dal-Pizzol, and J. Quevedo, "Methylphenidate Treatment Causes Oxidative Stress and Alters Energetic Metabolism in an Animal Model of Attention-Deficit Hyperactivity Disorder," *Acta Neuropsychiatrica* 26, no. 2 (April 2014): 96–103.

Chapter 33: Yarrow (*Achillea millefolium*)

1   M. Castleman, *The New Healing Herbs: The Ultimate Guide to Nature's Best Medicines* (New York: Bantam Books, 2002), 606.

2   J. A. Duke, *The Green Pharmacy* (Emmaus, PA: Rodale Press, 1997), 399.

3   Duke, *Green Pharmacy*, 53.

4   S. Yaeesh, Q. Jamal, A. U. Khan, and A. H. Gilani, "Studies on Hepatoprotective, Antispasmodic and Calcium Antagonist Activities of the Aqueous-Methanol Extract of *Achillea millefolium*," *Phytotherapy Research* 20, no. 7 (July 2006): 546–61, www.ncbi.nlm.nih.gov/pubmed/16619341.

5   S. Miranzadeh, M. Adib-Hajbaghery, L. Soleymanpoor, and M. Ehsani, "Effect of Adding the Herb *Achillea millefolium* on Mouthwash on Chemotherapy Induced Oral Mucositis in Cancer Patients: A Double-Blind, Randomized, Controlled Trial," *European Journal of Oncology Nursing* 19, no. 3 (June 2015): 207–13, www.ncbi.nlm.nih.gov/pubmed/25667123.

6   S. Pain, C. Altobelli, A. Boher, L. Cittadini, M. Favre-Mercuret, C. Gaillard, B. Sohm, B. Vogelgesang, and V. André-Frei, "Surface Rejuvenating Effect of *Achillea millefolium* Extract," *International Journal of Cosmetic Science* 33, no. 6 (December 2011): 535–42, www.ncbi.nlm.nih.gov/pubmed/21711463.

Resources

Other Books by Dr. Michelle Schoffro Cook

Boost Your Brain Power in 60 Seconds: The 4-Week Plan for a Sharper Mind, Better Memory, and Healthier Brain (Rodale)

The Probiotic Promise: Simple Steps to Heal Your Body from the Inside Out (Da Capo)

60 Seconds to Slim: Balance Your Body Chemistry to Burn Fat Fast (Rodale)

The Ultimate pH Solution: Balance Your Body Chemistry to Prevent Disease and Lose Weight (HarperCollins)

Weekend Wonder Detox: Quick Cleanses to Strengthen Your Body and Enhance Your Beauty (Da Capo)

Other Recommended Reading

Michael Castleman, *The New Healing Herbs* (Bantam Books, 2002)

James A. Duke, *The Green Pharmacy: The Ultimate Compendium of Natural Remedies from the World's Foremost Authority on Healing Herbs* (Rodale, 1997)

David Hoffman, *Medical Herbalism: The Science and Practice of Herbal Medicine* (Healing Arts Press, 2003)

Robert Rogers, *The Fungal Pharmacy: The Complete Guide to Medicinal Mushrooms and Lichens of North America* (North Atlantic, 2011)

Terry Willard, *Edible and Medicinal Plants of the Rocky Mountains and Neighbouring Territories* (Wild Rose College of Natural Medicine, 1992)

Herbal Supplies

There are a number of excellent companies that offer dried or bulk herbs for use in your herbal projects, particularly valuable if you can't grow all of your own. Two of my favorite suppliers follow:

Harmonic Arts
https://harmonicarts.ca/ref/65

Mountain Rose Herbs
http://www.mountainroseherbs.com/index.php?AID=133769

Acknowledgments

Thank you to the many wonderful people involved in making this book happen, specifically:

Georgia Hughes, Kristen Cashman, and the whole team at New World Library. You're a visionary group and a pleasure to work with.

Yarrow and Angela Willard, for your informative and entertaining herbal videos and blogs and excellent herbal products, and especially for your willingness to provide the foreword for this book.

Peggy Duke, for your botanical illustrations, which add beauty and a lovely energy to this book.

Jessica Kellner, Tabitha Alterman, Gina DeBacker, and the team at *Mother Earth Living* magazine for your support for my herbal column, which inspired this book.

My wonderful parents, Michael and Deborah Schoffro, for your ongoing support and belief in me.

Curtis Cook, my amazing husband and soulmate, for always treating me like a queen and supporting me in all that I do.

Index

stevia, 173, 180, 197
St. John's Day, 176
St. John's wort (*Hypericum perforatum*), 5, 13–14, 175–81
strep throat, 139
stroke-risk reducers, 89, 165
sulfur, 145
Sumerians, 78
superbug killers, 59, 89
Super-Healing Greek Salad, 142
Super Health-Boosting Pumpkin-Spice Latte, 61
Super-Simple and Delicious Black
Bean Chili, 52–53
sweating, 201–2
swelling treatment, 13
syrups, 11, 16, 191

Tabbouleh Salad, Gluten-Free,
146–47
tannin, 157
tarragon (*Artemisia dracunculus / Artemisia dracunculoides*), 134–35,
183–86
Tarragon Apricot Quinoa, 186
tea recipes: Anti-stress, 121;
Brain-Boosting, 173; Hor-
mone-Balancing, 162; Immune
Booster, 67; Mood Magic, 180–81;
Rosemary, 166; Smoking Cessa-
tion, 158; Stress-Soothing, 197;
Urinary Tract Healing, 102
teas, herbal, 11; clover, 161, 162;
dandelion, 57, 58–59, 60; echinacea, 67; horsetail, 95; how to make,
12–13; juniper, 102; lavender, 107;
lemon balm, 114; licorice, 121;
mint, 153; mullein, 129; peppermint, 151, 152; plantain, 158; rosemary, 166; sage, 171, 173; St. John's
wort, 180–81; thyme, 189, 190;
valerian, 196, 197; yarrow, 201

tendinitis, 133
testosterone, 165
Tex-Mex cuisine, 49
Thai Ginger-Coconut Soup, 91–92
throat relief, 44, 139, 187
thyme (*Thymus vulgaris*), 16, 167,
187–92
thymol, 187
thyroid support, 114
tinctures, 11; dandelion, 57; ginger,
90; how to make, 16–17; juniper,
101; lemon balm, 114–15; licorice,
119; oregano, 139, 140; plantain,
156; sage, 170; St. John's wort, 177;
tarragon, 184; valerian, 195, 196
tomatoes: Gluten-Free Tabbouleh
Salad, 146–47; Super-Healing
Greek Salad, 142
tonsillitis, 65
toothaches, 158, 185
toxicity, 11, 100, 101
toxins, environmental, 20
trichomoniasis, 130
triglycerides, 89, 126
Trojan War, 200
tuberculosis inhibitors, 72, 130
Tutankhamen (pharaoh), 118
Tylenol, 88

ulcer treatment: chamomile, 37–38;
licorice, 122; plantain, 158
United Kingdom, 132
United States Agriculture Department, 43, 78–79
urinary tract cleansers, 201
urinary tract infection treatments,
60, 101
Urology Journal, 146
U.S. Pharmacopoeia, 194

valerenic acid, 195
valerian (*Valeriana officinalis*), 112,
193–97

About the Author

Michelle Schoffro Cook, PhD, DNM, DHS, ROHP, is the author of eighteen health books, including the international bestsellers *60 Seconds to Slim, The Ultimate pH Solution,* and *The 4-Week Ultimate Body Detox Plan.* Her books have been translated into many languages, including Spanish, Greek, Chinese, Thai, Indonesian, and Russian. She holds advanced degrees in natural health, holistic and orthomolecular nutrition, and traditional natural medicine, and has twenty-five years of experience in the field. Dr. Cook is a board-certified doctor of natural medicine who has received the Doctor of Humanitarian Services designation from the World Organization of Natural Medicine and a World-Leading Intellectual Award for her contribution to natural medicine. She is a regular blogger for CulturedCook.com and Care2.com. Visit her websites DrMichelleCook.com and WorldsHealthiestDiet.com.

World's Healthiest News

You can subscribe to Dr. Cook's free e-zine, *World's Healthiest News,* to obtain natural health insights, news, research, recipes, and more.

Each edition features natural approaches to boost your energy, supercharge your immune system, and look and feel great. Subscribe at WorldsHealthiestDiet.com.

Dr. Cook's Blogs

Don't miss a single blog by Dr. Cook — follow her at:
DrMichelleCook.com
CulturedCook.com
HealthySurvivalist.com
Care2.com/GreenLiving/author/MCook

Discover Dr. Cook's exclusive e-books at:
WorldsHealthiestDiet.com

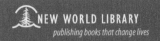